PRAISE FOR P1

It makes me wonder why more businesses and more employees/entrepreneurs don't focus more on these areas as a community where it would make the biggest impacts financially.

— INTERNATIONAL REVIEW OF BOOKS (STARRED REVIEW)

This little book just may have a big impact on the quality of your life.

— READERS' FAVOURITE (STARRED REVIEW)

I recommend *Peak Human Clock* to all readers that are working towards being fit and healthy.

— LITERARY TITAN (STARRED REVIEW)

Peak Human Clock is an insightful new guide to get you into your peak performance. Read this book! It will help you make smart decisions to optimize your life.

— SZE THO FOOK CHOONG, COO, UOB KAY HIAN

His information-filled self-help guide is especially recommended for readers who would not just increase productivity, but ultimately get their lives more in sync with their body's inherent system of wellbeing.

An intriguing but familiar glimpse into the mysteries of body clocks and sleep rhythms.

PEAK HUMAN CLOCK

HOW TO GET UP EARLY, FIX EATING TIME SCHEDULE, AND IMPROVE EXERCISE ROUTINES TO BE HIGHLY PRODUCTIVE

SAID HASYIM

Cover and Graphs
BARBARA BORKO

Sometimes taking time is actually a shortcut.

— HARUKI MURAKAMI

CONTENTS

INTRODUCTION

Have you ever wondered why you seem to be more alert at a specific time of the day? Or why you feel full of energy or lethargic at a particular time, or why you have the urge to go to sleep and wake up at certain hours? What if you could tap into this natural behavior of your body on every occasion and schedule your tasks around it to your advantage? Well, this is absolutely possible!

When you get your body's clock in tune, you can plan difficult tasks for when you are most alert, and complete them *faster* and at *double* the quality than when you perform them at other times of the day. Or you could plan to eat the junk food you have been craving during the hours it is less likely to be stored as fat in your body.

Jack, who is a hardworking white-collar worker, woke up at 7 a.m. to a jarring alarm clock. Still feeling sleepy, he resisted the temptation to snooze the clock and headed straight to take a shower. He then rushed to work and got a cup of coffee to stay awake. At noon, he went out for lunch and returned to the office at 1 p.m. While working on his computer, he felt sleepy, so he got another shot of coffee. It was Friday, and his friend invited him to go to a movie after work. He left work at 6 p.m., went out to dinner, and then joined his friends. He arrived home at 10:30 p.m. after the movie ended. Feeling hungry, he reached for donuts in his fridge. After satisfying his hunger, he scrolled through his friends' social media posts before hitting the sack at 1 a.m. He slept in the next day and woke up at 10 a.m. Still feeling tired, he continued to lie on his bed browsing videos on his phone before finally getting up at 11 a.m. to take a bath and eat brunch.

This is a typical day for Jack. He sleeps in on weekends and gets up earlier on working days. He is out of shape, feels sluggish most of the day, and after work, he has no motivation to do anything other than clinging to instant gratification. He has lost the energy he once had during his youth. Life goes on, and he thinks this is the reality of getting older.

Johnny, who is the same age as Jack, works in the same office as Jack. He understands the concepts of using his circadian body's clock. Every day, he wakes up at 6 a.m., exercises, and then has his breakfast before heading to the office. He is able to fully concentrate at work and does not feel sleepy during the day. To stay away from sluggishness in the afternoon, he drinks a spoonful of apple cider vinegar after lunch and goes for a short walk outdoors before returning to his desk. He eats his dinner at 4 p.m., and leaves the office at 6 p.m. After reaching home at 7 p.m., he learns one word in Spanish. He then winds down with relaxing music while reading his favorite book. As the clock hits 8 p.m., he meditates for ten to twenty minutes and goes to sleep. He follows the exact routine on the weekends. Instead of sleeping in on holiday, he works on his personal projects and hobbies.

Johnny always wakes up at about the same time every day and does not need coffee to get him through his productive hours. He is always in shape, rarely gets sick, acquires new knowledge daily, and is able to complete more things. What is his secret? He just honors his body's clock and does things at the right moment, when his circadian rhythm supports them. He forgoes many night events to get to bed on time. If he must stay up late for work, he wears blue light blocking glasses to prevent his melatonin from being suppressed.

I am going to show you specifically how to work with your circadian rhythm, so you can plan your days ahead and be more productive. I will walk you through, step by step, until you obtain the necessary information to get the outcomes you want.

Five years ago, after completing a Lean Six Sigma project, a data-driven approach for eliminating defects to streamline any processes, to help a company save time and money, I became obsessed with finding the best ways to maximize my productivity. I spent years doing a lot of research, performing self-experimentation, and bio-hacking with gadgets. I made adjustments to my routine, logged results every day to find correlations, and attempted to add an extra hour in a day by reducing the amount of time I slept at night. I discovered that working with your circadian rhythm is the best possible way to speedily increase your productivity and attain better physical and mental well-being.

As it turns out, we still function best the way ancient hunter-gatherers did. I took a considerable amount of time to fix my daily routines and set them aligned with my circadian rhythm, but the results are definitely worth the effort.

I know many friends and family members who face the same problems as Jack does. They work hard but don't feel productive during the day. They always hope tomorrow will be better.

I decided to write everything that I have learned throughout my journey to help them make changes to their lives forever. There are many methods to increase productivity, but this book focuses on implementing lifestyle changes that improve the functions of your body and brain by deliberately planning to execute your tasks at the ideal times, based on your body clock. The book aims to tackle the root of the issue within your own biology so you can carry the benefits with you permanently.

Getting to understand circadian rhythm is the first step in using it to your advantage.

1

CIRCADIAN CLOCK

> In the morning a man walks with his whole body; in the evening, only with his legs.
>
> — RALPH WALDO EMERSON

HAVING A DISRUPTED CIRCADIAN RHYTHM AFFECTS OUR productivity in many ways. We will look into what the circadian rhythm is, and the problems caused when our rhythm is out of tune.

I lived in Tanjung Balai Asahan, a small town in North Sumatra, Indonesia, when I was a young schoolboy. Every day, I woke up at 6 a.m., had a home-cooked breakfast, and I took a trishaw, a three-wheeled bike, to school. The ride took about fifteen minutes. Throughout the journey, I was exposed to morning sunlight. The school lessons ended by 1 p.m.

Afterwards, I headed home on a trishaw again and ate my lunch at home. Then I played outdoors with the neighborhood kids. Our games included hide and seek, rope jumping, and many more. When we finished playing, I took a shower to wash off the sweat and then ate dinner at 5 p.m. Afterwards, I spent time with my family until we went to sleep at 8 p.m.

I always had enormous energy as a young boy. I was ready to take on the day, did not get sleepy, had full concentration in class, always went to bed at 8 p.m., and woke up at 6 a.m. without an alarm clock. Heck, we didn't own an alarm clock even if we wanted to use one. There weren't many activities to do at night, and owning a phone was a luxury.

Entering into university life, I went to another country, Singapore, with a few friends of mine. I started to stay up late to finish school assignments. My friend introduced me to coffee as a stay-awake drink. I learned to snack on instant noodles or crackers when I got hungry at night. I woke up late on non-school days and sometimes joined my friends at parties until late at night. I felt more active at night and worn out during the day, thus I stayed most of the time indoors, except when I needed to go out to buy food.

Little did I know, I had disrupted my natural circadian rhythm, and caused it to run out of sync. The lifestyle I had adopted began to consume a lot of my potentially productive hours. How I wished I could go back to my younger self when I always felt powerful and prepared to face any challenges life might pose.

What is Circadian Rhythm?

So, let's examine the *Circadian Rhythm*, the natural 24-hour body clock operating throughout our body. We will discuss what it is and how it stops you from being productive when your clock is out of synchronization.

The circadian rhythm regulates all your body's organ clocks.[1] That's right! Every internal organ and function in your body has its clock. Your liver, lung, brain, immune system, heart, gut, saliva-generating glands, stomach, muscles, and pancreas all have their own clocks. At certain times of the day, each of them is programmed to tell the body when to ramp up the heart rate, digestion, strength, concentration, and melatonin production. They are all governed by a part of the brain called the Suprachiasmatic Nucleus (SCN).

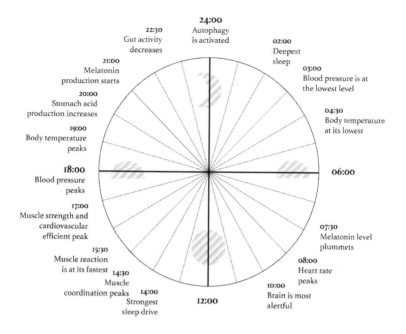

Circadian Rhythm

A healthy circadian rhythm looks like the preceding graph. When you wake up, the first light entering your eyes establishes the setpoint to reset your circadian clocks. Your cortisol (stress hormone) level increases to allow you to be awake and concurrently stops the production of melatonin. Your saliva production increases, and your digestive system is running at full speed, ready to process food. Your liver is prepared to absorb nutrients from the meal. Later in the morning, your brain clock and immunity system become more active.

In the afternoon, your sleep drive increases, something that is known as the afternoon slump, and you feel sluggish and sleepy. During the late afternoon, your muscle coordination and strength increase, readying your body to hunt.

Your body temperature peaks in the evening, and stomach acid secretion increases. Insulin response begins to slow down. Towards the late evening, your melatonin production starts to prepare your body to sleep, your body temperature cools down, and gut activity decreases to avoid having bowel movements when you sleep.

At night when you sleep, your body maintenance begins. Your salivary glands produce less saliva, your growth hormone increases, and as it gets closer to the morning, your cortisol level surges again.

This cycle repeats and resets every day, and if you maintain a healthy circadian rhythm, all your body's clocks will always run synchronously, allowing you to time your activities for best productivity.

Disrupted Circadian Rhythm

Having irregular routines in your life, such as an irregular sleeping schedule, disrupts your circadian rhythm as it develops confusion about what the correct time is, and attempts to reset itself every time you change your routine.

A chronically disrupted circadian rhythm causes a number of health problems, including:

1. Disrupted digestion

A disrupted body's clock throws off your metabolism rate, your digestion of fat and sugar, and your cholesterol. These may be more active at the time when you eat less and less active when you eat a lot. Consequently, you would increase your weight gain and be more prone to indigestion, constipation, bloating, and abdominal pain.

2. Increased inflammation

Your immune system thinks your body is under attack at all times and mobilizes its defensive mode again and again. This process causes inflammation, and your system is unable to regulate immunity well. Your susceptibility to viral or bacterial infection increases due to weaker natural defenses.

3. Increased risk of dread diseases

The kidney clock ensures your blood pressure goes down at night and up during the day. A disordered clock may keep blood pressure up during the day and the night, increasing the risk of a heart attack. A circadian misalignment also causes less healthy neurons to form up, which makes you less resilient against brain diseases.

4. Disarranged brain clock

Our brain does not correctly time the production of the hormone that regulates alertness and relaxation. As a result, you may not be alert at the time you should be alert, or relaxed when you should be relaxed. This increases your neuron stress and your anxiety.

5. Increased susceptibility to chronic stress

When your circadian rhythm is not in sync, your vulnerability to chronic stress increases. Chronic stress disrupts your circadian rhythm further. This creates a vicious cycle, and you need to break the cycle by tackling each of your body's clocks, one at a time, to slowly return to a healthier circadian rhythm. Furthermore, with cortisol production out of sync, your stress level is not well regulated.

6. Disrupted cells repairing

The bone-building process may not get turned on every day, which means your damaged cells or tissues are not getting cleaned up and regenerated on a timely basis. This leads to slower wound healing and weaker bones not being repaired.

YOUR CLOCK IS out of sync if you face any of these symptoms:

- You don't feel sleepy at a consistent time every night.
- Without an alarm clock, the time you wake up every day has more than an hour's difference than when you wake up with an alarm clock.
- You don't have regular bowel movements every day.
- You feel hungry at random times at night.
- You want to eat at night, even though you had just finished your dinner two hours ago.
- You wake up in the middle of the night and can't go back to sleep again.

All these things not only precipitate health problems but also ruin your productivity. Aside from giving you a list of health issues, it is impossible to plan your tasks optimally according to your circadian rhythm, because its clocks are not predictive.

Luckily, it is possible to get your circadian rhythm back in tune by setting up consistent *sleeping, eating,* and *exercising* routines.[2] Fixing these routines will get your body's clock back to normal.

IN THE NEXT CHAPTER, we will dig deeper into the first critical routine that we must fix: *sleep.*

2

MASTER YOUR SLEEP TO MASTER YOUR PERFORMANCE

> A night of sleep is as much preparation for the subsequent day's activity as it is recovery from that of the previous day.
>
> — J. ALLAN HOBSON

WAKEFIELD RESEARCH CONDUCTED A SURVEY IN 2018 AND concluded that more than 51% of the adult population worldwide is sleep-deprived.[1] In the U.S. alone, sleep deprivation contributes to about $411 billion of economic loss annually.[2] Work schedule, erratic lifestyle, uncontrolled screen time, and bad food choices are the biggest culprit of sleep deprivation. The impact is shocking, and I think people need increased awareness and proper education on sleep hygiene.

In this chapter, we will discuss how sleep helps your circadian clock be more robust, and how lack of sleep negatively impacts your performance. Then we will go into details on how to tackle sleep deprivation.

Sleep Helps with Circadian Rhythmicity

While research into the circadian clock is unraveling some intricate and amazing details, there is one thing that is pretty basic and entirely certain about our internal clocks. They like *routine* and *predictable* behavior. If you go to bed at the same time every night and wake up at the same time every morning, including weekends, your circadian clock will adapt to these times.

Deprived Sleep Deprives Productivity

Everyone knows how important sleep is, but how many put in the effort to make sure they get quality sleep? The single *most significant* contributing factor to your peak performance and mental clarity is sleep. Nothing beats a great night's sleep. Sadly, many underestimate the power of good sleep in the name of hard work and success. Most of the time, people sleep *less* during weekdays and sleep *more* on weekends and holidays to compensate for the sleepless weekdays. They don't have any regular, fixed sleeping schedule.

Depriving yourself of sleep results in a large number of problems, and you end up spending a lot more time on damage control.

1. Increased stress hormone production

Cortisol levels increase when your body does not get sufficient rest. If those levels are elevated over an extended period of time, the stress system becomes very sensitive. As a result, the brain overreacts to minor stressors. This also increases the risk factors for depression and makes you more irritable and prone to mood swings.

Regular sleep regulates your stress level throughout the day. Your cortisol level is higher as you wake up to prepare you for work and handling any stressful events, and lower at night to prepare you for sleep. When you have sufficient sleep, you also recover quickly from stressful experiences.

2. Reduced growth hormone production

The brain releases the growth hormone during deep sleep. This hormone is responsible for building muscle and increasing strength and exercise performance. Lower levels of growth hormone increase the risk of heart disease, obesity, and diabetes. Lack of sleep reduces the occurrence of deep sleep, which in turn reduces growth hormone production.

3. Decreased mental performance

Having just *one* night of poor sleep decreases your mental capacity, affecting decision-making and attention. Young children who sleep less perform worse at school than their peers who get enough sleep. Staying up late to review examination material reduces your performance during the examination the next day. You will experience brain fog and an inferior level of attention. Thus, it is much better to ensure you get sufficient sleep before your exams.

Every day, neural stem cells in the brain create new neurons. This generative process is called neurogenesis. The forming of new neurons enhances learning, motor skills, language acquisition, cognitive adaptation, and emotional control. Prolonged loss of sleep for just a week reduces neurogenesis. This causes your cognitive function, attention, and long-term memory to weaken. The brain starts to be more forgetful and face difficulties storing any memories.

Furthermore, a lack of sleep increases your fatigue during the day, which reduces your cognitive functions. Fatigue causes you to make more mistakes, blunts your workout progress, and makes you less active, which encourages your body to deposit excess energy as fat.

4. Increased risk of chronic diseases and mortality

Lack of sleep causes the most *accidents* in the world. Sleep deprivation also increases the chance of dying from all causes, especially cardiovascular disease, heart attack, heart failure, stroke, and diabetes. The Centers for Disease Control and Prevention (CDC) in the United States estimated that the risk of death caused by insufficient sleep is up to 13%.[3]

As the number of hours you sleep decreases, your blood glucose levels increase, and your insulin sensitivity drops. Just one week of being sleep-deprived raises your blood glucose level to a dangerously pre-diabetic level.

Sleep deprivation also decreases the body's ability to repair damaged cells and slows the repair processes our body needs. Our body recycles its bad cells with new cells through a process called autophagy. This process is necessary to boost the immune system and protect against disease. Autophagy is activated several hours after the last meal, which often occurs when you are asleep. When you don't sleep enough, autophagy activity slows down. By giving yourself sufficient sleep, your body is able to replace more defective cells.

Sleep helps fight inflammation. When you are sleep-deprived, you are more prone to illness because your defense system does not have sufficient time to put off the inflammation.

5. Increased risk of obesity

Insufficient sleep reduces the time your body spends burning fat. Your body starts using fat for energy about eight to fourteen hours after your last food intake, with the majority of the time spent burning fat being during sleep since that is the longest block of time in a day without food. If you deprive yourself of sleep, you have a higher tendency to snack before bed, which reduces the chance for the body to burn fat.

Sleep deprivation disrupts your hunger and satiety hormone production. When your stomach is hungry, it produces Ghrelin, the hunger hormone. This hormone is vital because it makes you feel hungry. On the contrary, Leptin is the satiety hormone produced when you are full and signals the brain to stop eating.

Its production increases during sleep so you don't feel hungry, as there is plenty of energy available in fat storage.

The production of the ghrelin hormone decreases during sleep, which explains why you are not hungry while sleeping. When you are sleep-deprived, your ghrelin and leptin hormones are not in alignment. Lack of sleep decreases leptin and increases ghrelin, so even though you might have just had a big meal, the imbalance of these hormones leads to overeating. The worst part is that your appetite for salty or sweet food increases.

On top of that, in a sleep-deprived state, your brain prefers instant gratification and therefore triggers your craving for energy-dense food. Coupled with the decrease in willpower, this often results in sweet or caloric-dense food bingeing, leading to obesity. This is an important negative setback if you are on a strict diet. Additionally, when you don't get enough shut-eye, the number of microbes in your gut that promote obesity increases. All of these build up the tendency to gain fat.

So, not only do you lose productivity if you are sleep-deprived, but there are also a number of health problems to deal with. How much sleep do you need, then?

How Long Should You Sleep?

To reap all the benefits of sleep, you may think more is better, but sleep can have adverse effects when it is *overdone*. A study conducted by the American Heart Association shows that oversleeping, which is defined as sleeping for more than ten hours for adults, increases mortality, and death by cardiovascular disease.[4]

The table below serves as the guideline for the duration of sleep needed by different age groups.

Sleep Duration
(Hours)

0–3 Months	14-17
4–11 Months	12-15
1–2 Years	11-14
3–5 Years	10-13
6–13 Years	9-11
14-17 Years	8-10
18-64 Years	7-9
>65 Years	7-8

Required Amount of Sleep

Source: Hirshkowitz, M. et al. (2015). National Sleep Foundation's sleep time duration recommendations: methodology and results summary. Sleep Health, 1(1), 40–43. https://doi.org/10.1016/j.sleh.2014.12.010

It should be noted that the time here refers to the time you sleep, not the time in bed. You may stay in the bed for ten hours, but you are not really sleeping if most of the time you are tossing around in your bed.

Do not attempt to wake up earlier than your body needs for the purpose of gaining additional hours in your days.You do indeed get to use the additional hour(s), but you are screwing up your productivity with lowered cognitive functions and sleepiness during your waking hours.

During my years of experiments, I tried to extend my days by waking up very early. I would go to bed by 8:30 p.m. and wake up by 4:00 a.m. At that time, I did not have my sleep quality fixed yet, so while I was in bed for seven and a half hours, I might only have been sleeping for less than six hours. I was able to maintain my wake-up time at around 4:00 a.m. every day, but I did not get the results I wanted. I had extra hours, but I noticed that my performance suffered, and I mostly felt sleepy during the day.

When you sleep less than what your body requires, you accumulate sleep debt. Let's assume you need eight hours of sleep daily, and you only clocked in seven hours last night. This means you have one hour of sleep debt. On a subsequent day, you sleep for eight hours, but you still have that one hour of sleep debt. When you have accrued a significant sleep debt, your body will attempt to recover it the next night by falling asleep earlier or waking up at a later time the following day.

Ideally, you should find ways to keep your sleep pattern as consistent as possible, but as we know, sometimes life gets in the way. If there is any sleep debt, allow your body the chance to recuperate the following night by going to sleep earlier, waking up later, or taking a nap.

Oversleeping on weekends does not compensate for five sleep-deprived workdays. It is not possible to clear all sleep debt in one or two weekends, not when you sleep too little for an entire workweek. Your body operates on a 24-hour circadian clock. It will not allow you to enter a rejuvenating sleep when the time is not right according to your body's clock. Do not accumulate a lot of sleep debt. Help your body to clear them as much as possible the following night and get back to your regular sleeping schedule.

Monitor your sleep time and note how many hours you need to function well each day. We are all different, so keep in mind that the amount of sleep varies depending on your activities that day. If you do an intense workout, you will need to sleep one to two hours longer that night to allow your tired muscles to recover.

It is downright possible to cut down the amount of sleep every night if you can increase your sleep quality.[5] Sleep quality *trumps* sleep quantity. Let's discuss what you can do to improve your sleep quality and finally get in sync with your circadian rhythm, starting with understanding the different stages of sleep.

Sleep Stages

In effect, we all know that we do not instantly fall asleep, because our brain does not shut down as soon as we lay our heads on a pillow. Instead, our brain takes time to progress through the various phases. Understanding how your body and brain function during sleep allows you to be aware of its importance, so let's take a closer look at the stages of sleep.

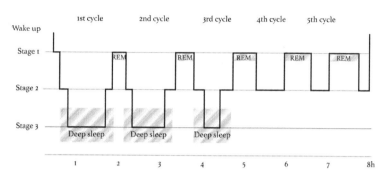

Sleep Stages

STAGE 1

At first, our brain prepares to drift off and experiences periods similar to daydreaming, but here we are starting to doze off. We begin to enter a brief period where we linger between being awake and asleep. However, we can still perceive things around us and maintain a sense of awareness. An average sleeper takes about seven minutes to fall asleep, but you may fall asleep slower or faster.

This is a shallow, choppy sleep, and in this stage, any disturbance can wake you up with ease. We spend about 5% of the night in this stage, and it occurs in blocks that continue for 1–7 minutes.

STAGE 2

Our brain starts to produce very short periods of rapid, rhythmic brainwave activity. Body temperature begins dropping, and the heart rate starts slowing.

Your body then releases the Human Growth Hormone (HGH), which helps to develop muscle tissue. At this stage, we are not as easy to wake up as when we are at stage 1. We settle about 45% of the night in this phase, and we stay in it for blocks that last 10–25 minutes.

STAGE 3

Stage 3 is a transitional period between light sleep and REM (Rapid Eye Movement) sleep and is often called deep sleep. This is the *most* restorative stage of sleep. During this period, it is difficult to wake you up, and any interruption that wakes you up while in this stage will make you feel very unstable for a while.

The pressure of your blood drops at this stage. More HGH is released to grow muscle and accelerate repair. Blood supply to muscle increases, the body repairs itself, builds bones, grows tissues, and improves the immune system.

We spend about 25% of the night in this stage, and we remain in it for blocks of 20–40 minutes.

STAGE 4

This stage is known as REM (Rapid Eye Movement) sleep. At this stage, your eyes move back and forth fast. Dreams occur at this moment, and your body paralyzes your muscles to avoid any movement when you are dreaming; your blood pressure and heart rate increase. Sleepwalking and bed-wetting may happen at the end of this phase.

The brain consolidates memory at this stage, and transfers short-term memory to long-term memory storage, allowing you to store new information. When awakened at this moment, you will feel groggy and very sleepy. The first block of REM sleep is shorter, and they get longer as cycles repeat. At this period, lactic acid built up during exercise, which causes muscle soreness, is broken down, and your body heals any minor muscle tears.

We spend around 25% of the sleep in this stage, in blocks of 10–60 minutes. One cycle of sleep is complete when you move from stage 1 to stage 4, with each cycle lasting about ninety minutes. Stage 3 lasts longer during the first sleep cycle and gradually lasts for shorter periods of time towards the end of the sleep. The *inverse* applies to the REM stage, which lasts for shorter periods of time during the initial sleep cycle and then gradually lasts longer towards the end.

When you wake up too early, you sacrifice REM sleep duration, and when you are interrupted during your sleep, you likely sacrifice deep sleep (stage 3) duration.

HIGH-QUALITY SLEEP CONSTITUTES UNINTERRUPTED SLEEP, sufficient sleep duration, and the right amount of deep and REM sleep. As each stage of sleep restores different functions of our body, it is vital that you don't skip any of the stages and that you get undisturbed sleep at night to allow adequate sleep time and reap all its benefits.

Sleep Tracker

If you always have problems with sleep, I suggest that you invest in a sleep tracker when you are trying to improve your sleep. Having a tracking device helps you reach your goal faster. The tracker allows you to view your sleeping pattern, waking-up pattern, and discover any issues you are not aware of, as well as how long your actual sleep time is and how long you are in the REM and deep sleep states.

Having this information allows you to make adjustments for better sleep. Maybe you will realize that you often wake up at a particular hour of the night due to noise from the neighbors, or that you can sleep better with a ten-minute meditation right before sleeping when compared to doing it an hour before sleeping. Gaining some insights into your sleeping habit and behaviors makes it possible for you to form your plan to eliminate the root causes.

There are many sleep trackers in the market now, ranging from wearable devices to non-wearable devices. If you don't like the idea of wearing a wristband while you sleep, you can get a non-wearable device which is installed under the mattress or clipped on the pillow. Some trackers even include a wake-up function to wake you up when it detects that you are at the lightest stage of sleep during your preset wake-up time window. This helps you avoid waking up in the wrong stage.

Fix Your Sleeping Schedule

We will start with fixing your sleeping schedule, followed by tips to gain quality sleep.

Let's begin by adjusting the sleep schedule and ensuring consistency. Sleeping at a regular time every day may be a luxury for people who must work on a shift schedule that varies weekly. I am sad to say that it is impossible to train your body's clock when you keep changing your sleep time.

If you are lucky and don't need to keep altering your sleeping schedule for work, the following steps will help you fix a new sleeping routine.

Set your ideal sleeping time and follow it daily, including weekends. It's going to take a lot of willpower to maintain consistency. Bear with me for this long journey. Once you complete this hard part, you will embrace your natural sleep-wake cycle time.

1. Adjust fifteen minutes weekly

If your perfect sleeping time is much earlier than your current one, adjust your current sleeping time by fifteen minutes every week until you reach your desired time. Be patient; it is going to take a while because you cannot, in an instant, tweak your body's clock to wake you up at a certain hour. Give it time and keep a consistent and predictable behavior for your clock to reset to the new rhythm.

Strive to wake up five to ten minutes before your set wake-up time, then decrease it every week towards your target time. The earlier you wake up, the earlier your body will want to get you to sleep to achieve the total sleep duration needed.

2. Exposure to morning light

Get your morning sunlight exposure for about ten to twenty minutes when you arise to reset your circadian clock in the morning. Try to aim for the light to hit the lower part of your eyes. It is as if having the light shining from the top of your head. Get your daily dose of sunlight before 10:00 a.m., because after that time, the ultraviolet radiation is at its strongest, which is harmful to your skin.

If your wake-up time is before sunrise, your body's reaction will be different. The darkness gives your brain the signal that it is *not yet* time to get up. In such a case, use a bright light therapy device to signal the body that it is daytime, and tell your body and brain that you should be awake so it should stop producing melatonin. There are plenty of bright light therapy devices available, including portable ones. They prove to be very useful if you need to adapt to waking up pre-sunrise.

Such devices are also handy when you don't have time to get sunlight outdoors upon waking up due to indoor tasks that need your immediate attention.

Studies show that your susceptibility to blue light, which affects your melatonin production at night, decreases when you expose yourself to bright light during the day.[6] Furthermore, bright light exposure during daytime improves melatonin secretion in the evening and improves your mood and attention, getting you energized and ready to face the rest of the day.

3. Increase sleep drive

Your body starts accumulating the drive to sleep when you wake up in the morning. Every waking hour adds thirty minutes to sleep drive, and when it peaks, you will feel a heavy burden to sleep. Manipulating the variables below can help to adjust your sleep drive:

- An afternoon nap *decreases* your sleep drive. Avoid afternoon naps unless you have sleep debt. If you must take a nap to recover some of your sleep debt, do not sleep for longer than forty-five minutes. Longer naps decrease your sleep drive further, and you will likely push your sleeping time even later that night.
- Physical activity *increases* your sleep drive and melatonin production in the evening, so get yourself some exercise to sleep better.
- Caffeine *decreases* your sleep drive. Avoid coffee and chocolate past noon, since chocolate contains caffeine as well. Caffeine can stay in your system for ten hours, so if you need to consume it, take it as early as possible in the day.

4. Melatonin supplement

Melatonin is a hormone responsible for making you feel sleepy. Your brain secretes melatonin at night according to your usual sleeping schedule. It starts producing melatonin between two and four hours prior to your normal bedtime. As we age, the production of melatonin decreases, which is why older people often have trouble going to sleep.

If it is difficult for you to sleep earlier than usual, consume melatonin supplements about two hours before your expected bedtime to help you start sleeping earlier. Always start with the lowest dose possible and observe how your body reacts to it. A higher dose of the supplement can cause grogginess, a headache, and nausea during the day. Everybody does not respond the same way; for some, 0.1 mg is enough to aid in sleeping, but for others, they need as much as 5 mg to experience any effect.

At present, there is no evidence that long term use of melatonin is harmful or creates an addiction. Until further research provides more information, to be on the safe side, avoid using it for two weeks in a row to lessen the possibility of your body adjusting its natural melatonin production to accommodate for its artificial increase.

Do not take melatonin right after your dinner, because it slows the process of lowering the blood glucose level back to the normal level.[7] Blood glucose goes back to the base range within one to two hours after a meal. You can take melatonin afterward, in order not to interfere with the blood glucose regulation.

Consuming a melatonin supplement should be treated as the last resort when you have trouble adjusting to a new schedule or if you are having difficulty falling asleep but there is an important event the next day that you need to attend to. It is always best to rely on the body's natural melatonin secretion.

Fix the Sleeping Environment

Making adjustments to your sleeping environment helps increase your sleep quality.

1. Get rid of noise pollution

If you live in a place that is always noisy, or you work shifts and need to sleep when the rest of the world is awake, then the quality of your sleep will be impacted by the noise. Below, you will find a few options for tackling the problem of noise pollution.

- **Bedroom soundproofing:** This is done by installing a door sweep at the bottom of your door to cover the gap, installing thick curtains to absorb the sound coming from the windows, mounting bookshelves or hanging pictures on the walls to add some thickness to the walls, installing weatherstrip tape on the windows and door, or installing carpet to absorb noise from the floor. It may not be possible for some people to get all these done in their bedrooms because of the decor or limited furniture. However, if you can apply most of them, it will help reduce the noise considerably.

- **Earplugs:** The next option is to wear a pair of earplugs to sleep. These should block all sources of noise, including your snoring sleeping partner. However, it is inconvenient for some to wear earplugs while they are sleeping. Some people complain that they are painful for their ears during sleep and after waking up.
- **Over-the-ear speaker headphones:** The alternative to earplugs is over-the-ear speaker headphones that play white noise to mask other noises. The headphones can be placed over the ears instead of in the ears, which makes them easier to bear.
- **White noise machine:** If you don't like to wear anything at all to sleep, a white noise machine is the best choice. It is a machine I bring with me every time I travel. White noise machines emit a constant loop of sound to mask possible noises that could occur throughout the night. If you are using an audio file to play white noise instead, make sure to set it to play in an endless loop without you being able to detect when the music ends and repeats. The sudden stop and start of the machine could wake you up if you are a light sleeper.

2. Reduce your core body temperature

Core body temperature refers to the temperature of the internal environment of our body, which includes organs and blood. Our internal temperature starts to cool down at night in preparation for sleep. The dropping temperature serves as the

cue to get to sleep, while an increase in temperature is the cue
to wake up.

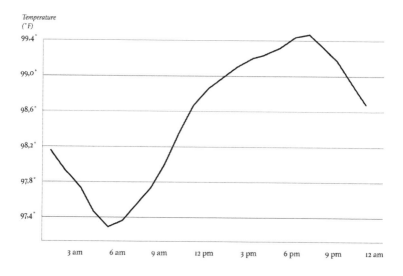

Body Core Temperature Throughout the Day

When you are sleeping, your core body temperature goes down
by 0.9 °F to 1.8 °F (0.5 °C to 1 °C). By purposely dropping your
core body temperature, you can trick your body into sleep
mode. A few ways to do so are as follows:

- **Cool sleeping environment:** An air conditioner is
  useful for keeping the bedroom cool. Since our body
  temperature changes throughout the sleep cycle, you
  don't want to wake up in the midst of the night feeling
  too hot or too cold. Finding the right temperature that
  suits you requires trial and error, and testing a range of
  temperatures. Spend some time to experiment with
  setting the air conditioner to turn off or change the
  temperature at certain hours during the night to get

uninterrupted sleep and not be woken up to increase or decrease the temperature. If your air conditioner has no function to perform the temperature adjustment automatically, you can install an infrared (IR) controller that can be programmed to adjust the temperature of the IR-controlled air conditioner unit at certain times of the night. If you sleep with a partner who has a different preference for a sleep temperature, you may consider setting up a cooling mattress system which is capable of maintaining two different temperature zones, one on each side of the bed. While using an air conditioner is an indispensable option in tropical countries, it dries the air in the room, causing your throat to be dried when sleeping. Installing a humidifier solves this problem. Alternatively, if your bedroom is not large, having a wide container filled with water is sufficient.

- **Take a warm bath:** A warm bath or shower before bed increases your body temperature, but when you are done and get into your cool room, your body will feel cool and experience a drop in temperature. This signals the brain that it is time to sleep.
- **Wear socks:** Many research studies concluded that wearing socks to sleep shortens the time it takes to fall asleep.[8] Wearing socks warms up your feet and causes the heat to escape from the skin, which, in turn, lowers your core body temperature. Be sure to choose soft and breathable socks instead of compression socks, so your feet do not get too warm while sleeping.

3. Complete darkness

Smartphones, computers, electronic devices, LED lamps, even a lowly dimmed light, emit blue light. Blue light exposure near bedtime suppresses melatonin production, which makes you fall asleep later, decreases your REM sleep, and delays your circadian rhythm. These outcomes are the opposite of the objective you want to achieve when you are trying to sleep. As much as possible, avoid blue light in the evening. Disorders of the sleeping rhythm often start with blue light disturbance.

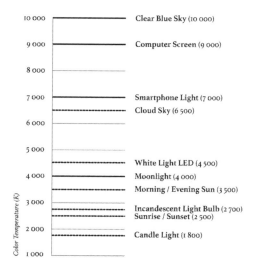

Color Temperature

Candlelight (<2,000 K) is an excellent choice as it emits almost no blue light. There are commercially available LED bulbs that do not emit blue light, too, although they are more expensive than regular LED bulbs. Replace your lamps with blue light blocking bulbs if you can.

If you can't avoid blue light near your bedtime or it is impractical to replace all your house lamps with low blue light bulbs, wear blue light blocking glasses with lenses that block out blue light and stop your brain from becoming overstimulated by it. Choose one that blocks 100% of the blue light wavelengths from 450 nm to 510 nm. These are the most harmful wavelengths, and not all blue light blocking glasses can protect 100% against blue light at this range. Wear them for one to two hours before your bedtime to encourage melatonin secretion.

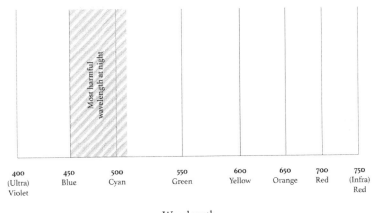

Wavelength

When you go to sleep, ensure that your bedroom is dark without any trace of light. Even the tiniest level of light entering your eyes lessens melatonin production. Blackout curtains or blinds are helpful to protect against external light sources. Cover all LED lights on any electronic devices in your bedroom, such as the LED panel from an air conditioner, with black stickers. If you cannot seal all possible sources of light, wear a mask to sleep.

Wear the blue light blocking glasses if you wake up at night to go to the toilet. It helps to guard your eyes against the blue light exposure if you need to switch on the light or if there is any source of light on your way to the toilet. Exposure to blue light at this stage makes it difficult to go back to sleep afterward.[9] This is very apparent for people with severe insomnia.

4. Bedroom association

Your brain needs to tell your body that your bedroom is a safe place to raise your parasympathetic tone, which aids your attempts to sleep. If you often experience stressful situations in your bedroom, your brain will make the association that it is a stressful environment and then activate more sympathetic tone, causing you to have difficulty falling asleep. Design and arrange your bedroom solely for the purpose of sleep and romance instead of using it to reply to hectic emails or watch disturbing news and movies. Make it your perfect sanctuary for sleeping and do not use it for entertainment or work.

Note: Our autonomic nervous system has two divisions: the sympathetic nervous system and the parasympathetic nervous system. The sympathetic nervous system triggers the "fight or flight" response in the brain when it detects that you are in danger, and adrenaline surges through your body to help you run away or attack. The parasympathetic nervous system does the opposite by triggering a "rest and digest" response after the danger is gone.

Both are useful for different situations, and your brain toggles them on and off to support your survival. When the parasympathetic nervous system becomes active, the sympathetic nervous system shuts down, and vice versa. Chronically activating the sympathetic nervous system raises your cortisol hormone constantly, making you suffer from chronic stress. Contrarily, activating the parasympathetic nervous system too much increases the risk of mania.

5. Sleeping partner

Having a sleeping partner, like a spouse, a kid, or even a pet, may disrupt your sleep. A snore or movement of your spouse, or a kick delivered by your kid while dreaming can wake you up. Sleep alone, if possible, but if you can't, use separate blankets to help isolate movement.

6. Scent

For generations, people have used scents for healing purposes. Scents can play a role in helping you sleep better, as well. Lavender, vanilla, and bergamot scents promote sleep. Chamomile, lemongrass, lemon, and orange smells induce calmness.

Studies discovered that the scent of lavender supports deep sleep.[10] There is no shortage of commercial products that can help you with this, such as an aroma diffuser, a sleeping mask cream, or a pillow spray.

7. Air purifier

Studies showed that improving the quality of the air improves the quality of your sleep.[11] Install an air purifier or get plants that purify the air. NASA research approved Snake Plant (Sansevieria trifasciata) as an excellent air purifier. This plant not only removes toxins from the air but also converts carbon-dioxide to oxygen during the night, making it ideal for keeping it in the bedroom.

8. Red light

A red light in the evening stimulates the production of melatonin and increases sleep quality.[12] It does the opposite of what blue light does to melatonin. Replace your evening lamp with a red light to increase your melatonin production before bed. If you are not used to sleeping in complete darkness, you can also sleep with a red light on.

IT WOULD BE best if you can apply all of these, but if you can't, or it is impractical for you, don't be discouraged. Once you have already experienced good sleep quality using some of the methods, applying more improvements gives you diminishing returns.

Finally, keep a sleep journal to determine what needs adjustment, and create your own individualized blueprint for the best sleep. Everyone's body responds in different ways. Track some events that you think contribute to your sleep quality and make adjustments based on those. Your tracking could include:

- The time of your last large water intake.
- When your last meal was.
- Whether you got sunlight in the morning.
- When you wore the blue light blocker glasses.
- What the intensity of your exercise was.
- Whether there were any stressful meetings in the afternoon.
- What the air conditioner temperature was.
- What you did before sleeping.

When You Cannot Sleep

Even after fixing everything you can, there will likely be times when you still can't sleep at night. Maybe you had a stressful meeting earlier, or you have a troubling situation, or your mind is racing about tomorrow's big event. So, let's examine what you can do when you have problems falling asleep.

Typical advice includes listening to music, reading a book, listening to an audio-book, journaling, and drinking hot milk. These are all good suggestions, and if they are effective for you, that's excellent.

Based on my personal experience, some of these are not practical for me.

For example, regarding reading a book, you should grab one that is not very exciting or one that does not require you to think too hard. Arousing your brain at this hour will trigger cortisol secretion.

Drinking hot milk is not suitable for people who practice intermittent fasting and end their last meal hours before bedtime, as I do. Furthermore, the goal is to avoid food intake close to bedtime.

After experimenting with many other options, I found two things that work for me every time:

1. **Slow breathing exercise:** Breathe in slowly for four seconds, hold your breath for seven seconds, and breathe out for eight seconds. Doing so lowers your resting heart rate, which activates your parasympathetic tone, and you force your mind to focus on your breath instead of something you may be worried about. Inhaling activates your sympathetic tone, while exhaling activates your parasympathetic tone. Practice lengthening the duration of your exhale to increase parasympathetic stimulation. This method is straightforward to apply as you can do it on the bed itself, which makes it my first choice.
2. **Melatonin:** Always try the first method before resorting to consuming melatonin. Be mindful of blue light on the way to take the melatonin supplement. Consuming a melatonin supplement will bring you to sleep fast. I usually go with this option when I am stressed, and my brain is still racing even after meditation.

You can apply these two methods to fall asleep fast without sacrificing precious time doing other activities or breaking your fast with a glass of milk.

YOU SHOULD SEE a marked difference in the quality of your sleep if you make the changes laid out previously. With many people in the world not having appropriate sleep hygiene, the amount of effort and time it takes to cure the long-term illnesses it causes is enormous. If you want to function at your best, and build a robust circadian rhythm, make good quality sleep your *priority* in life.

In the next chapter, we will discuss the next routine that helps you fine-tune your circadian rhythm: *exercise*.

3

WE ARE BORN TO MOVE

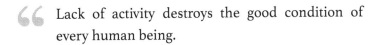 Lack of activity destroys the good condition of every human being.

— PLATO

GLOBALLY, 60% TO 85% OF ADULTS LIVE A SEDENTARY lifestyle.[1] A sedentary lifestyle is a global health problem and the leading cause of death and disease. Most people know that exercise is essential for their well-being, but they are often not motivated to get into the habit of exercising because they don't see results right away. Exercise has to be part of your routine to promote the synchronization of circadian clocks.[2]

In this chapter, we will analyze how exercise helps with your productivity, and its other numerous supporting benefits, the types of exercise you should prefer, and the fundamental requirements for muscle gains.

Role of Exercise in Productivity

Studies have proven that exercise can increase your productivity by 21%.[3] The performance boost is mainly attributed to improved energy and mood, increased brain-derived neurotrophic factor (BDNF), and increased willpower.

ENERGY AND MOOD

Our body still operates the same way it did hundreds of thousands of years ago when hunter-gatherers went out to hunt animals for food and stored fat to last for the moments of food shortage. If your lifestyle is sedentary, your body does not think that you will need much energy (to hunt), and it encourages fat storage, thinking that it is probably not the hunting season yet, and you will need food reserves.

We only have limited energy in a day, and when we are low on energy, we feel tired and are unable to concentrate on working. Everything we do produces low-quality results. This is a waste. Having high energy all day long allows you to accomplish more things and be more productive. Extraordinary results require much energy, and exercise begets more energy.

Exercising is a means to increase your mood and destress your body. Dopamine, norepinephrine, and serotonin are released when you exercise. These neurotransmitters stimulate feel-good chemicals in your brain to regulate and improve your mood for the rest of the day.

Repeatedly stressing your body without overdoing it makes your body more efficient at recovering from it. Regular exercise makes you more resistant to stressful situations. The effect is not permanent, and the stress resistance tapers off if you quit exercising.

BDNF

BDNF is the brain-derived neurotrophic factor that is produced by your brain to help existing brain cells survive. It repairs injured neurons and stimulates the growth of new neurons and synapses in a process called neurogenesis. Maintaining high levels of BDNF allows effortless learning and high retention of memories. Reduced levels of BDNF results in problems with memorizing and difficulty in learning.

The best way to increase BDNF production in the brain is consistent exercise, aside from having good quality sleep and restricted caloric intake.

Not all exercises induce the same level of BDNF increase:

- Anaerobic exercise does not increase BDNF.[4]
- Intense anaerobic exercise, in which you complete the repetitions to failure, increases BDNF.[5]
- Aerobic exercise increases BDNF, but an intense aerobic exercise of about 80% of maximum heart rate exertion increases BDNF the most.

Note: Completing repetitions to failure means performing the exercise to the point of momentary muscular failure, in which case you won't be able to carry out any further repetitions in a given set.

WILLPOWER

Willpower is the currency of the maximum tasks you can do in a day. Without us realizing it, we are tapping into our willpower with everything we do daily, whether it is important or not important. Deciding which clothes to wear? We drain our willpower. Solving a complex problem? We drain more willpower.

Regular physical exercise is one way to build up your willpower. It takes a tremendous amount of willpower to build a habit to exercise. Once you form an exercise as a habit, and it becomes an enjoyable experience for you, it won't take much willpower to exercise. It is no wonder that most people who exercise regularly lead better lives, partly due to their high willpower. I have detailed the strategies to optimize willpower in another book, *Peak Self-Control*.

Notable Health Benefits

You either spend your time developing good health now or spend your time and money on healthcare. Aside from the performance improvement gained from exercise, there are numerous health benefits exercise provides that could help you stay away from hospitals.

1. Improved heart function

Resting heart rate is the number of times your heart beats when you are resting. It is best measured first thing in the morning before you perform any activity. Having a high resting heart rate indicates poor physical fitness. Your heart is not efficient and needs to beat more times to do its job. If your heart beats seventy times per minute, that is 100,800 times a day, and 36,792,000 times a year. Hearts grow weaker as we age. If you want your heart to function longer, take care of your heart to reduce its resting rate. Exercise is the most effective way to reduce your resting heart rate and improve cardiovascular health.

Age	18-25	26-35	36-45	46-55	56-65	>65
Athlete	49-55	49-54	50-56	50-57	51-56	50-55
Excellent	56-61	55-61	57-62	58-63	57-61	56-61
Good	62-65	62-65	63-66	64-67	62-67	62-65
Above Average	66-69	66-70	67-70	68-71	68-71	66-69
Average	70-73	71-74	71-75	72-76	72-75	70-73
Below Average	74-81	75-81	76-82	77-83	76-81	74-79
Poor	>82	>82	>83	>84	>82	>80

Men's Resting Heart Rate

Age	18-25	26-35	36-45	46-55	56-65	>65
Athlete	54-60	54-59	54-59	54-60	54-59	54-59
Excellent	61-65	60-64	60-64	61-65	60-64	60-64
Good	66-69	65-68	65-69	66-69	65-68	65-68
Above Average	70-73	69-72	70-73	70-73	69-73	69-72
Average	74-78	73-76	74-78	74-77	74-77	73-76
Below Average	79-84	77-82	79-84	78-83	78-83	77-84
Poor	>85	>83	>85	>84	>84	>84

Women's Resting Heart Rate

Source: Alessi, G. (n.d.). Give my heart a break - resting heart rate. Core Principles. https://www.coreprinciples.com.au/ online-personal-trainer2/item/give-my-heart-a-break- resting-heart-rate.html

2. Increased muscle mass

Strength training increases muscle mass, which helps burn more calories when you are at rest, reduces the body fat percentage, and makes you leaner. Having more muscle mass also protects you against age-related muscle loss, called sarcopenia.

3. Increased bone strength

Use it or lose it. When we don't use our bones, the body has no incentive to keep them strong. Any exercise that stresses the bones, such as strength training, promotes the growth of more durable and denser bones. Having strong bones is essential to prevent fractures as we get older. A sedentary lifestyle degrades bone mass, but strength training helps slow down age-related bone loss.

4. Balanced blood sugar level

After demanding physical activities, your muscles are hungry to soak up a good amount of glucose from the blood. This helps reduce the sugar level circulating in your blood, and the chance of developing insulin resistance.

Note: Insulin resistance occurs when your cells resist the signals from the insulin secreted by the pancreas, ordering them to shuttle glucose from the bloodstream into cells. As a consequence, the glucose builds up in your bloodstream and leads to a high blood sugar level. As your body is unable to use the glucose for energy, it gets stored as fat.

5. Reduced evening cortisol levels

Cortisol levels subside in the evening. However, people who exercise have more significant reductions in their cortisol levels in the evening, which is very useful in preparing you for better sleep at night. [6]

Types of Exercise

In general, you could perform two types of exercise: *aerobic* and *anaerobic*. Aerobic exercise such as jogging and bike riding requires oxygen to keep up with the workout steadily for a longer period of time. Aerobic exercise gives a boost to your cardiovascular health and metabolism. Your body will perform better with regular cardio sessions. But, as the name suggests, the cardio workout is aimed at making your heart healthier.

Long aerobic training helps your body with metabolic adaptation. Muscles become more efficient in absorbing available glucose in your system and learn to tap into fat stores for energy when there is no more glycogen available.

Note: Glycogen, made from the glucose in food, is the fuel used for exercise. Your body converts the carbohydrate you eat in the food into glucose. When your body does not need to use glucose soon, it is converted to glycogen and stored in the liver and muscle.

In opposition, anaerobic exercise has higher oxygen demands, and your body can't sustain the workout for long. An example of anaerobic exercise is strength training or resistance training. Performing anaerobic exercises helps to build muscle over time. Every time you stress your body with anaerobic exercise, your body strengthens your muscles to handle the stress better next time. It is this muscle adaptation mechanism that helps you get fitter and stronger.

Some women are afraid to do strength training because they worry they will pack their bodies with bulging muscles. This is far from the truth because women just do not produce as much testosterone as men, so they cannot build up their bodies to look like Arnold Schwarzenegger.

When Can You Start Exercising?

Starting at the age of three, children can safely perform any light aerobic exercise. Being physically active at an early age helps them grow stronger bones, keep obesity at bay, increase strength, and maintain an active lifestyle as they grow up.

Careful consideration, however, has to be done for young children to start strength training:

- If they are less than twelve years old, allow them to perform only bodyweight exercises such as squats, push-ups, or sit-ups. Supervise them to ensure they perform the exercise with correct form.
- If they are thirteen years old, they may start strength training with light weights, to avoid the risk of injury.
- If they are fifteen years old, they can lift a little heavier weight since their bones are stronger now.
- If they are more than eighteen years old, they can start lifting heavy weights because all the body functions have finally developed in full. It is easier for adult men at the age of 17–25 to bulk up due to the high level of growth hormone, which starts to decline between the age of twenty-five and thirty. That is why youngsters can pack muscle on faster when compared to older people.

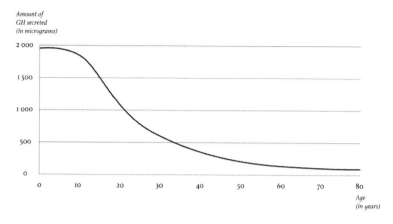

Growth Hormone Secretion by Age

There is no scientific evidence that strength training in young children stunts their growth. However, any injury caused by strength training will, indeed, hamper their growth if they do not perform the exercises with the right form. Proper execution of the technique will work fine and not harm the child's growth.

The Basics of Strength Training

Building an effective strength training program requires that you take the *frequency* of training, the *order* of the exercises, and the *rest period* between sets into consideration. A good workout program is not one that's too long, as it is counterproductive; working out for too long increases cortisol and lowers testosterone. A good workout length is between forty-five to sixty minutes.

Consider the efficient order of the exercises to maximize their effectiveness. Plan to prioritize *compound (multi-joint) exercises* before *isolation (single-joint) exercises.* This way, you can ensure that you have enough energy to work out multiple parts of your muscles in the beginning. An example of this kind of strategy is that you shouldn't work out abs and biceps first. Fatigued abs won't be able to protect your back when you do back exercises, and fatigued biceps can't help you with other exercises that use biceps secondarily.

There are many good strength training programs developed by fitness experts available in books or online. If you are a beginner, I recommend that you read *Starting Strength* by Mark Rippetoe, and if you are an experienced lifter, I recommend reading *The M.A.X. Muscle Plan* by Brad Schoenfeld.

Some useful terms used in strength training:

1. Repetitions

Lower repetition programs in strength training, with 4–6 reps with a heavy load, are good for building strength; moderate repetitions, 8–12 reps with a moderate load are good for muscle growth (hypertrophy); higher repetitions, 15–20 reps with lighter loads are good for building endurance. Strength training requires that you rest for 3–5 minutes after every set, while endurance training requires that you rest for less than thirty seconds or as short as possible after every set.

When you are training for hypertrophy, you will have a moderate rest period of 60–90 seconds. If your goal is to gain muscle, it is important that you also train for strength and endurance. Strength training allows you to lift more weight over time and to build fast-twitch muscle fibers, while good endurance allows you to lift at higher intensities with little rest and to build slow-twitch muscle fibers.

	Repetition	Load	Rest Time
Strength	4 – 6	Heavy	3 – 5 mins
Hypertrophy	8 - 12	Moderate	60 – 90 secs
Endurance	15 - 20	Light	< 30 secs

Training for Strength, Hypertrophy, and Endurance

Note: There are two main groups of muscle category: slow-twitch (type I) muscle fibers and fast-twitch (type II) muscle fibers. Your body uses slow-twitch muscle fibers first to meet the demands of the exercise. When slow-twitch muscle fibers cannot cope with the force that's required, your body will then use fast-twitch muscle fibers.

Fast-twitch muscle fibers are activated the most when you train for strength by lifting heavier weights with low repetitions. In contrast, slow-twitch muscle fibers are activated the most when you train for endurance by lifting lighter weight with high repetitions. Fast-twitch muscle fibers produce more force but fatigue faster than slow-twitch muscle fibers. That is why you need a longer rest time to recover between sets when you train for strength and less recovery time when you train for endurance, as your slow-twitch muscle fibers would have recovered, making you ready to lift in the next set.

2. Weight

Pick a weight that you can lift with perfect form. If you use a program that requires you to do 12–15 reps, the weight is too heavy for you if you can't do at least twelve repetitions, and too light if you can do more than fifteen repetitions with perfect form.

3. Technique

Resistance training is not about getting from point A to point B. You need to contract the muscle. Because you are training the muscle, ensure that you always use the proper technique or form. Don't rush to complete the workout and thereby sacrifice form. It is not a race to lift as fast as possible. Use the correct tempo of the exercise.

In general, perform concentric moves (lifting the weight up or positive phase) as explosively as possible, and eccentric moves (lower lift or negative phase) slowly to maximize muscle and strength gain. The technique to lower the weight is equally important as lifting the weight.

Delayed Onset Muscle Soreness (DOMS) is the soreness in your muscles after working out. It results more from eccentric movement than concentric movement.[7] Don't short-change the eccentric movement. For every exercise you want to perform, research the instruction on how to do it beforehand.

4. Breathing

People often overlook the breathing technique during weight training. Proper breath techniques help you work out harder. Exhale on concentric moves, and inhale on eccentric moves. When lifting heavy weights, we tend to hold our breath slightly longer to push through the movement, but when overdone, you may pass out due to lack of oxygen flowing to your brain.

Exercise Fuel

It is vital that you fuel your workout to amplify its effectiveness. Please note that this is a general workout meal plan for your daily workout, and not intended to be a meal plan for a sports race or competition.

Pre-workout meal

Before your workout, aim to include complex fibrous carbohydrates in your meal. Complex carbohydrates release glucose into your system gradually. This will give you a steady supply of energy to fuel your workout later. Don't eat a heavy meal too soon before working out. If you do, your muscles will compete for the oxygen your body needs to digest the food. Aim to eat about one and a half hours before your workout.

About fifteen minutes before working out, consume fast-acting protein such as whey to reduce muscle breakdown and increase protein synthesis after a workout. At this point, avoid fatty foods because they slow digestion. Your energy shall be maximised for your workout instead of digestion while you are working out. This is not the case for coconut oil because it is absorbed and used by the body fast.

If you work out first thing in the morning, do you still need to consume carbohydrates? That depends. On an average person, the muscle can hold about 300 grams of glycogen, which is enough for a little less than one hour of intense running. People who do strength training and are on a high-carbohydrate diet are able to store 900 grams of muscle glycogen.

After your overnight sleep, your body would have depleted the glycogen in your muscle and liver to a certain degree. Your muscle glycogen will still be able to supply energy for your workout if it is not too intense. Once you've emptied your muscle glycogen, your body will trigger gluconeogenesis, the process of converting the stored glycogen from the liver into glucose to fuel the workout. This process is slow and inefficient for strength training.

Your body will probably still be able to power through a moderate intensity workout, but if your workout is intense, you will empty your muscle glycogen in no time, and the body will resort to gluconeogenesis. In such a case, consuming carbohydrates prior to your workout is beneficial to your strength training.

If you strength-train fasted, it will increase your muscle breakdown, and you will be losing muscle over time. To prevent that, consume Branched-Chain Amino Acid (BCAA) supplements beforehand to minimize muscle breakdown.

PERI-WORKOUT (DURING WORKOUT) MEAL

A peri-workout meal is optional. Some people find having a peri-workout meal inconvenient. If you consume a peri-workout meal, you will probably go with one in liquid form as it would be difficult to eat solid food while working out. Consuming fast-acting protein at this point is advantageous to kick-start muscle recovery.

When you sweat during a workout, you lose water along with electrolytes, which contains potassium, chloride, and sodium. If you practice intermittent fasting and you are very active, re-hydrating your body with water that is mixed with Himalayan Pink Salt nourishes your body with over eighty-four minerals. Mix a half-gallon of water with a quarter teaspoon of Himalayan Pink Salt as your peri-workout drink. If you do not fast and are not a very active individual, your regular meals throughout the day should have sufficient salt intake, and you don't need to add extra salt into your total food intake.

POST-WORKOUT MEAL

Our body is at its peak to absorb nutrients about one hour after working out. It is not necessary to expeditiously consume a post-workout meal within one hour if you had a pre-workout meal already.[8] If you train fasted, consuming a post-workout meal soon is good to halt muscle breakdown or catabolism. Take the information below into consideration when deciding when and what to consume for your post-workout meal:

- Research showed that a combination of carbohydrates and protein results in higher protein synthesis for muscle repair and growth.[9] The high Glycemic Index (GI) carbohydrates help create high amounts of insulin to synthesize protein. This means ingesting high GI carbohydrates after a workout regenerates glycogen at a faster rate compared to consuming carbohydrates hours after a workout.[10] You can consume carbohydrates and protein at a ratio of 3:1. If you are not going to work out again in the next twelve hours, consuming high GI carbs right after exercise is not compulsory, because your glycogen synthesis will be fully stocked through the next twenty-four hours.

Note: The Glycemic Index, or GI, is the measure of how much the food can affect a person's glucose level. High GI food, such as sweet potatoes, fruit juice, and white bread, causes glucose levels to spike, while low GI food, like non-starchy vegetables, is absorbed at a slower pace and does not spike the blood sugar level.

- Avoid fast food, which adds fat to your body and slows digestion. You need the protein and glucose to get to your muscles as quickly as possible.
- Fibers slow digestion, so you should avoid high fiber food right after a workout if you want to maximize protein synthesis. You can eat high fiber food about an hour after your post-workout meal.
- When selecting fruit to replenish muscle glycogen, avoid fruits that are high in fructose, which only replenishes liver glycogen and not muscle glycogen.

You can, however, choose fruits that contain high glucose to fructose ratio, such as the banana. High glucose to fructose ratio means the amount of glucose is higher than the amount of fructose in the fruit. The good thing about consuming fruits after a workout is that they contain a lot of vitamins, minerals, and possibly antioxidants that help the tired body.

	Glucose per 100g	Fructose per 100g	Glucose to Fructose Ratio
Grapes	6.5	7.6	0.85
Blueberries	3.5	3.6	0.97
Pomegranate	5	4.7	1.06
Kiwi	5	4.3	1.16
Sweet Cherries	8.1	6.2	1.3
Figs	3.7	2.8	1.32
Banana	4.2	2.7	1.55

Glucose to Fructose Ratio

Foundations to Gain Muscle

Strength training is your arsenal to build muscles. Aerobic training can increase muscle size only on untrained individuals who have not received any training stimulus. Let's check some components that you should note when your goal is to gain muscle.

1. Progressive overload

You will notice your body composition will change when you start strength training, but over time, your body will adapt to the exercises you perform. Growth will be very slow or even halted because your body will have gotten used to the exercise. Alter your exercise program to shock your muscles with different workout routines. A common mistake of weightlifters is following the same program routine for too long.

Training with the same weights every session will not grow the muscles beyond a point. Your muscles will become accustomed to the monotonous weight, and thus there will be no need to develop bigger. Increasing intensity through the added weight, volume, or lower rest time puts stress on your muscles and stimulates growth.

2. Rest

Your body needs a rest day to recover from intense workouts. Your muscles build when you are resting. You don't have to do six workout days and one rest day; you could plan the exercise according to muscle groups targeted in each session. As an example, avoid hitting the same muscle group back-to-back the next day. With proper nutrition, major muscle groups require up to four days to recuperate. Muscles will not grow if there is insufficient time for the tissue to repair itself.

Working out lays a foundation for building muscle. Good quality sleep is what does the muscle-building, coupled with nutritious food intake. We looked at the importance of sleep earlier in the book, and it is vital for your muscle-building regime. A lack of sleep when trying to build muscle undermines all the hard work you are putting in at the gym. Aim for 7–9 hours of sleep. Muscle grows during the deep stages of your sleep when your body produces high levels of growth hormone.

An intense workout program with sufficient rest days yields better results than having fewer to no rest days. During your rest days, do some active recovery exercises such as light cardio, biking, or swimming. This helps flush out lactic acids from your muscles and reduce soreness. Incorporate cold showers to enhance muscle recovery.

3. Training Frequency

How much do you need to work out to continue gaining muscle, while keeping the gains proportional to the extra effort? After the initial gains on untrained individuals, the rate of muscle growth declines. Undoubtedly, people who spend a lot of time working out may be making better gains, but you will need to consider whether you are willing to put the additional 60% of effort in just to get 4% of the gains while increasing the risk of overtraining. If you are an elite athlete, you may need to do that to get past the growth ceiling, with the necessary monitoring of your recovery status to avoid the pit of overtraining.

Several research studies show that low-frequency training does not necessarily mean no gain.[11] Training the same muscle group twice a week works great to increase muscle mass.

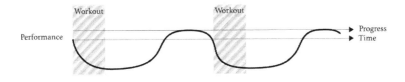

Training Too Infrequently

When you train too infrequently, your body takes too long before it receives the next stimulus and loses the opportunity to grow.

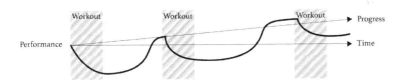

Training at an Optimal Frequency

When you train right after your body has recovered, you grow stronger, and compound muscle growth over time.

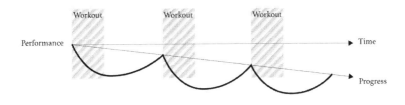

Training Too Frequently

Source: Zatsiorsky, V. M., Kraemer, W. J., & Fry, A. C. (2020). Science and Practice of Strength Training (Third ed.). Human Kinetics, Inc.

When you train too often, your body does not sufficiently recover before the subsequent session, causing it to get fatigued over time, before it has a chance to adapt and grow stronger.

Training too frequently leads to overreaching and ultimately overtraining. Overreaching is the state your body gets in when you continue to train in an under-recovered state. Your body feels a temporary loss of strength after an intense workout session. Every once in a while, implementing a program that allows overreaching is essential to deliver a higher stimulus for muscle growth. Still, it should be followed by deloading week(s) when you train at a lower intensity and less frequency. Continuing to ignore the symptoms of overreaching leads to a more severe problem: overtraining.

Overtraining occurs when your body continues to endure the state of being under-recovered. It is unable to catch up with recovery anymore, your cortisol level stays elevated even at rest, and your body perceives it as chronic stress, which causes higher inflammation levels. Your body needs to repair not only your muscles but also your central nervous system. Aside from losing your motivation to train, it will take months, if not a year or so, to recover enough to return to your original state.

Overreaching   Overtraining

- Mild sleep disruption
- Temporary reduced performance
- Temporary fatigue
- Temporary muscle soreness
- Temporary increased heart rate
- Temporary increased frequency of colds

- Chronic sleep disruption
- Disturbed mood
- Reduced performance
- Chronic fatigue
- Chronic muscle soreness
- Slow recovery
- Increased heart rate
- Frequent colds
- Loss of motivation
- Lower testosterone
- Chronically elevated cortisol levels
- Loss of appetite

Symptoms of Overreaching and Overtraining

Each body recovers at a different rate, with many factors affecting the speed and effectiveness of the recovery, such as sleep quality, diet, and stress level. How can you figure out your optimal training frequency to maximize the effect of your training? Most advanced athletes track Heart Rate Variability (HRV), which is a reliable way to monitor recovery before hitting the pit of overtraining. Several HRV tracking devices on the market are highly accurate. Using these devices allows you to take the guesswork out of the equation while maximizing your exercise response by planning its frequency based around your HRV.

Note: The Heart Rate Variability is a measure of variation in the time interval between each heartbeat. A higher HRV means your body is recovering well and is capable of handling stress. At a high HRV, your resting heart rate is lower, and you can handle stressful situations when they arise. A lower HRV means your body is taxed. There is less variation, and your body stays at a high resting heart rate. When your HRV reading is high, you are ready to hit the gym, and when it is low, it indicates you need more rest.

4. Strength training over aerobic exercise

If you are planning to do aerobic exercises and strength training in the same session, always perform strength training first before the aerobic exercise. You want to maximize your strength training performance using your glycogen store and not depleting it in the aerobic exercises first. Remember that strength training is anabolic, which means it can only use carbohydrates, while aerobic exercise can use both carbohydrates and fat for fuel.

Limit your endurance training to up to two times per week if your primary goal is muscle-building. Endurance training inhibits muscle growth and deteriorates strength due to the different pathway adaptations it activates.[12] Strength training activates the mTOR (mammalian Target of Rapamycin) pathway, which is responsible for muscle growth and tissue repair. In contrast, endurance training activates AMPK (AMP-Activated Protein Kinase), which is responsible for breaking down glucose, fatty acids, and amino acids. Frequent AMPK pathway activation inhibits the mTOR pathway, slowing your muscle gain goal.

5. Macronutrients

To build muscle, you need to consume more calories than you expend. This will create a calorie surplus, and the extra calories can be used for muscle-building when you sleep. If you practice intermittent fasting, it is going to be hard to eat at a calorie surplus because you tend to eat less, though not impossible.

To know if you are in a calorie surplus, you need to know your maintenance calories, the number of calories required to maintain your current weight. If you are serious about muscle-building, this is one daunting task you need to work on. Without knowing your maintenance calories, nor tracking your meals, you are prone to consume too much surplus that would lead to being overweight. Eat about 15% more calories than your maintenance calories. Don't increase your calorie intake too much, as you will gain fat faster as well.

Computing your maintenance calories is individualized. There are many things to take into consideration, such as your basal metabolic rate, and activity level. There is no fixed formula to get an exact number out of this, as everyone is different. Many websites offer to compute the estimated calories needed, which you can do for free. Plan your macronutrient intake at the ratio of about 50% carbohydrates, 30% protein, and 20% fat for muscle gain.

Protein synthesis caps at around 25–30 grams per meal. Thus, it is best to spread protein intake throughout several meals in a day to maximize your muscle protein synthesis.

As a start, you will need to get some help to determine the macronutrient content of the foods you are consuming. There are some applications available that could help you with this. It is a really tedious task computing the calories and measuring the macronutrients every time you eat. However, as you become more aware of the macronutrient composition of the foods you always eat and you start to develop a consistent daily food plan, you may no longer need to measure the calories and macronutrients religiously.

6. Calorie cycling

Introduce calorie cycling into your routine. Consume more calories on your workout days, and lower calories on your non-workout days. Doing this allows you to be in a calorie surplus on your workout day to build muscle while keeping your calorie intake moderate on your non-workout day to avoid excess calories.

After strength training, your muscle-building potential heightens and then tapers off depending on your body response and age. The growth potential ends after about two days.

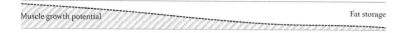

High-Calorie Surplus All the Time

When you consume at a high-calorie surplus daily, your body uses the extra calories for muscle-building after your strength training session, and over time a continuously rising surplus of calories is stored as fat.

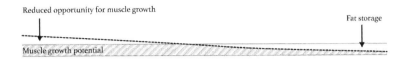

Low-Calorie All the Time

If you always eat at a very low calorie, worrying that you will gain fat, you miss the opportunity for muscle growth, and you gain a little fat on your rest day as well.

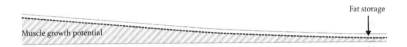

High-Calorie Surplus and Gradually Lower Calorie

But if you manage to consume at a high-calorie surplus around your strength training sessions and a smaller calorie surplus on your rest days, you not only maximize your muscle growth but also minimize fat storage.

Consume most of your carbohydrates around your workout to fuel your workout and recovery. Your body will partition the carbohydrates directly for workout fuel and recovery instead of fat storage, also known as carb-tapering.[13]

7. Keep a journal

Keeping a journal of your workout ensures that you can track your progress, and it serves as a system for you to measure your improvement. You can't improve on something that isn't measured. Track at least the number of sets and reps performed, and the weight used to set the baseline for your next workout and to know if you are progressing or have stopped progressing (reached a plateau).

The equation for muscle growth is adequate protein + calorie surplus + progressive overload + adequate recovery.

If you have halted your progress, change the following variables:

- **Add a rest day(s):** The problem is often that your body is overworked. Adding rest day(s) gives your body more time to recuperate and come back stronger.
- **Increase your calorie intake:** Your progress could be halted because of insufficient calorie intake, causing your muscles to stop growing. Aim for sufficient protein intake, too.
- **Fix your form:** Check if you have been completing the exercises with the correct form. Trying to use heavier weights before you are ready will compromise your form. Do not increase the weights if your form is incorrect.
- **Change your exercise program:** Sticking to the same exercise program for too long causes your body to adapt to it over time, which slows your progress. Change your program every 1–3 months to give your body new stimuli.
- **Sleep more:** Insufficient sleep blunts your muscle growth. Give your body 7–9 hours of sleep to have enough time to rebuild muscle tissue and help restore your central nervous system to give you the extra push.

ON THE WHOLE, exercise is your way to better productivity. Aside from helping you function better, it improves the synchronization of your circadian rhythm.[14]

Exercise should be formed as a lifestyle instead of a temporary endeavor just to gain certain benefits. Your mind and body work well when you do regular exercise. The benefits of exercise wear off a few weeks after you stop exercising.

Next, we will discuss changes in *eating* habits to fine-tune our clocks.

4

EAT HOW WE ATE

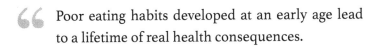 Poor eating habits developed at an early age lead to a lifetime of real health consequences.

— Richard Codey

Based on a 2016 statistic from WHO, the World Health Organization, about 39% of the world's adult population is overweight, and 13% are obese.[1] Studies show that overweight and obese workers cause substantial direct and indirect productivity losses as a result of sick leave taken, medical costs, disabilities, and mortality.[2] A random eating lifestyle is the primary cause of obesity and being overweight.

We will look into the problems with a random eating lifestyle, the importance of time-restricted eating, and how this type of eating pattern helps you lose weight.

Problems with a Random Eating Lifestyle

In this modern life, most of us focus more on what we put into our mouths and not on when we do it. On a working day, we sometimes skip breakfast or have it on-the-go while commuting to the office. After returning home from work, we have our dinner and then grab a jar of almonds and snack on them while watching TV. On weekends, we wake up later and eat our breakfast closer to the afternoon, and then have a late dinner. On some days, when we need to catch an early morning plane, we eat way earlier than our usual breakfast time. If you always eat at random times, you throw your digestion clock out of sync. You deprive it of food when it is optimized to process food, and you force it to digest food during times when it is less efficient.

This is an example of the type of random eating patterns most people practice. Your stomach does not know when to anticipate food or when to go into maintenance mode after you have stopped eating for the day. On random nights, when your stomach has finished processing food to prepare for repair, you surprise it by eating cookies. Your pancreas is not prepared to secrete insulin at that time, which means there is only a low level of insulin available to bring glucose into muscle cells. This condition leaves you with a high blood glucose level in your bloodstream. Your stomach is caught off-guard, and it must force itself to handle this unexpected emergency food while it is busy repairing your digestion system. Your digestive system now needs to drop whatever it is doing and start directing its attention to digesting food. Since the stomach is not prepared to process the food, it will take longer to complete the digestion.

Your body starts to burn fat about 8–14 hours after your last meal depending on the type and amount of food you eat. By the time it is about to tap into your fat storage for energy, it is going to be morning, and you may already be getting ready to eat breakfast. As a result, your body has no or only a brief period of time to use your body fat.

The body is also flooded with glucose from the carbohydrates or proteins from the food most of the time, making your liver less efficient in absorbing glucose, which increases the risk of diabetes.

If you have been eating at random times every day and snacking through the night, chances are you have been suffering from acid reflux, heartburn, a weaker immune system, poor sleep quality, irregular bowel movements, obesity, insulin resistance, indigestion, joint pain, and fatigue. Perhaps you have been dealing with these problems for so long that they have become ordinary parts of your life; you think it is just a typical experience of getting older.

Time-Restricted Eating

Intermittent fasting is a way of eating in which you alternate periods of fasting and feasting. By scheduling fasting into your eating plan, you give your digestive system a break and detoxify your body from the chemical-laden food that is difficult to avoid in this modern life.

Primitive humans did not possess the luxury of having their meals served three or four times a day. They hunted, feasted, and hibernated as needed. There were times when there was no food to hunt, and they needed to intermittently fast until they could find food. It wasn't until the post-industrial age that we had plenty of food from mass production. As an abundance of food was available to most people, they neglected proper eating habits. We overeat even when we are not hungry, and our digestive system has to work harder than ever to process the constant inflow of food.

There are a few types of intermittent fasting:

- Fast for twelve hours, and feast for twelve hours every day, also known as *Time-Restricted Eating.*
- Fast for twenty-four hours every other day, also known as *Alternate-Day Fasting.*
- Fast for twenty hours, and feast for four hours every day, also known as *Warrior Fasting.*
- And probably many more.

Of all the fasting methods, I strongly suggest time-restricted eating for at least twelve hours every day, starting and ending the fast at the exact hour, to regulate your circadian clocks with consistent feeding and fasting time. For example, if your first meal is at 6:00 a.m., complete your last meal at 6:00 p.m. if you are fasting for twelve hours.

Keep the timing as consistent as possible to influence your body's clock. Your body will learn to expect food at certain times and activate all the necessary digestive functions. Your stomach will know when to end food processing and kick-start maintenance mode during the fasting hours.

The first meal signals the body to start metabolic processing, and the end of the last meal signals the body to switch back to maintenance mode. After the last meal, the body needs to be entirely sure there is no more incoming food before turning on the repairing process. If you maintain the consistent last meal timing, your body will adjust to the schedule fast.

Take your time to adjust the fasting period to be longer if you wish, up to sixteen hours. Dr. Satchin Panda did a lot of studies with mice on the benefits of time-restricted eating in his book, *The Circadian Code*.[3] Incorporating this type of eating pattern into your lifestyle is easy. You can keep it consistent without having to decide which days to do intermittent fasting.

There are many benefits of performing intermittent fasting:

1. Body fat reduction

Intermittent fasting allows your body to use fat for energy. When you are in a fasted state, your body depletes the glucose in your blood, and it begins to tap into your fat storage for fuel when there is very little glucose left. When you are in a fed state, your body will not need to tap on your fat reserve.

Fasting also reduces the pressure to store fat. When you keep eating at any moment, your pancreas is encouraged to keep producing insulin, which inhibits fat breakdown and triggers fat deposits. Your body will not tap into the fat storage; it will instead continue to use the glucose from your blood.

If you go for an extended period without eating, the fat-storing capacity tapers down, and your body starts to use fat for energy. It also increases your insulin sensitivity, which allows the sugar in your blood to be normalized and used more effectively. With higher insulin sensitivity, your body is more efficient in shuttling the sugar to muscle cells instead of depositing it as fat. As the amount of fat reduces in your muscle cells and liver, it frees up room for more glycogen storage, which helps reduce sugar levels in your blood.

Many people worry about losing muscle mass when they practice intermittent fasting. The University of Illinois at Chicago conducted a study to measure the muscle mass loss of obese men and women after eight weeks of alternate-day fasting.[4] At the end of the eight weeks, the study concluded that no loss of muscle mass had occurred from alternate-day fasting. Muscle loss occurs only after about three days of not eating.

If you practice time-restricted eating at consistent times, your body will adjust your hunger and satiety hormone. During the beginning, when you start practicing fasting, you will notice signs of hunger after your last meal, but as you become adapted to this eating pattern, the hunger pangs lessen. Your brain becomes accustomed to feeling hungry at the time when it expects food and not feeling hungry after your last meal, as long as you consume enough calories for the day. This allows you to control your food intake better.

Studies also show that fasting increases the secretion of Human Growth Hormone (HGH), which is useful for the maintenance of muscle and bone and boosting exercise performance.[5] HGH deficiency leads to higher levels of body fat and a decrease in bone mass.

2. Sleep improvement

Time-restricted eating makes your body's clock more robust. As you always start your first meal and end your last meal at the exact time, your digestive organs become better synchronized to your eating time, which helps your body be more consistent with your sleep schedule.

When the last meal is two or more hours before bedtime, your digestive system rests and is not active, which calms your body for a better and deeper sleep.

3. Gut microbiome balancing

We own trillions of microbiomes in our gut that flourish or die when we are fasting or feasting. Having different numbers of microbiomes is essential to protect your body from inflammation, heal intestinal walls, fight disease, and regulate stress response. Without diverse microbiomes inhabiting our gut, we cannot completely digest our food, resulting in fat storage.

To increase the diversity of microbiomes in your gut, you need to eat a variety of food, or take probiotics, or practice intermittent fasting. Studies show that fasting suppresses the harmful microbiomes that promote obesity while helping good microbiomes flourish, which helps to better absorb the nutrients in our food and reduce cholesterol levels by metabolizing the bile acid produced in the liver.

4. Lifespan increase

There are countless research studies conducted which show fasting slows down aging.[6] Incorporating intermittent fasting in your routine may expand your lifespan. Numerous studies also show that intermittent fasting wards off chronic diseases since it reduces inflammation.

Every time we eat, we bring bacteria into our bodies. Our immune system needs to be activated to combat these invaders. This response to the invaders by our immune system is called inflammation. When you eat too often without giving your body enough of a food break, you acutely elevate the inflammation. Fasting reduces inflammation in your body as it is given a break from fighting the bacteria. With fewer inflammatory agents entering the body, the immune system has an increased capacity for repair and recovery.

Research indicated that fasting for at least fourteen hours every day, for twelve weeks, reduces cholesterol levels.[7] If you suffer from high cholesterol now, practicing time-restricted eating is your natural remedy for lowering the marker.

Autophagy is the process of recycling dead or damaged cells in the body to produce new cells; it is essential in the protection against cancer, inflammation, aging, insulin resistance, and neurodegenerative diseases. Autophagy is less active during feasting and more active during fasting. Its process begins to initiate when your glycogen level is low in the liver, that is, about fourteen hours after your last meal. Fasting enhances this function.

Fasting also strengthens the connection between brain cells, called neuroplasticity, which gives you better cognitive function, learning, and memory.[8] With the increase of neuroplasticity, brain injuries can be healed faster, which reduces the chance of neurodegenerative diseases.

Guide to a Time-Restricted Eating Lifestyle

Anyone from as young as five years old can practice time-restricted eating to prevent obesity and other problems associated with random eating times. Start your time-restricted eating journey now with the following steps:

1. Define the suitable first and last mealtime

Start by deciding first and last mealtimes that you can follow every day, including weekends. It is often easy to stray from the schedule on the weekend. Time them in accordance with your workout times, too, so that you can consume your heaviest meal after your workout session. It is not optimal to start a workout session after your last meal or deprive your body of the nutrients it needs the most post-workout. It is also not ideal to have your strength training session before your first meal because you will not have sufficient fuel to maximize your strength training.

Time your last meal at least 2–3 hours before your bedtime to ensure it does not interfere with your sleep. You want to obtain the benefits of both fasting and good sleep. Favor having your last meal as early as possible. We have learned that our digestive functions do not work as efficiently after sunset as they do during daytime.

Breaking the fast in the afternoon is easier for most people because we could make use of the sleeping hours to add to the duration of the fasting. The downside is that you will end up eating too heavy into the late evening. If this time fits you well, please go with it. Doing so is still much more beneficial compared to a random eating pattern. On a side note, consuming a carbohydrate-heavy meal in the evening helps reduce your stress level.

2. Start with a shorter fasting time

Start with 12-hour fasting, and after two weeks, or when you feel comfortable with your fasting schedule, transition to longer fasting periods if you wish. Most people have no problem practicing 12-hour fasting. If you try starting with a long fasting period, or end your last meal too early, fighting to stick to this fasting regimen will exhaust your willpower. As a result, you may face intensified temptation to quit before giving your body enough time to adapt and realize the benefits of fasting. Don't rush to get quick results if you cannot maintain the fasting protocol for life.

What constitutes breaking the fast? There are many definitions of what breaks the fast, with some defining ingesting zero-calorie food such as coffee or tea as not breaking the fast, while others consider that any food breaks it. In the context of giving a total break to the circadian system and kick-starting its revitalization process, any food except water and medicine breaks the fast.

Black coffee has zero calories and is acceptable in many intermittent fasting protocols as a beverage that does not break the fast. Having coffee enter your system still triggers the digestive clock to start secreting gastric juices, and the liver clock to start metabolizing the caffeine. This does not give total rest to your system if your purpose is full detoxification. However, if your goal is to eat fewer calories for weight loss, consuming zero-calorie foods during the fasting period will serve it well. If your doctor prescribes you any medicine, please continue to consume it. Medicine is not considered food.

3. Ensure sufficient caloric intake

Make sure you eat and drink enough. During fasting, drinking a lot of water is important to flush the bad cells, as they are replaced, out of the system. Water is the perfect medium for this. It passes through the body fast and takes these damaged cells with it on the way through.

If you are currently eating three meals per day, stick to eating the same three meals per day, but keep those meals within the hours allotted for eating. Do not reduce the number of meals because you are eager to lose weight fast. It can be quite tempting to skip a meal as you may not feel hungry when it is time to eat your last meal, which you used to eat later, nevertheless, you should try to eat it.

The focus here is not to create a calorie deficit, but to train and align your body to the new eating pattern and fine-tune your circadian rhythm. Losing some pounds by doing this alone is possible without changing your calorie intake.

If you reduce your calorie intake while adapting to time-restricted eating, you will be hungry at night. This will tax your willpower and inevitably increase the chances that you will quit this practice. As you are venturing into this good new habit, do not let this minor temptation stop your journey.

4. Adjust to your perfect time

When you are starting this change, your body is not yet familiar with the new timing, and you may not be able to accurately gauge the food intake that you are consuming throughout the day. It is also possible that you find it hard to eat a heavy meal in one sitting at the specific feeding time, or you might feel better having the heaviest meal as your last meal, so please adjust your first and last meal according to your preference. You want this new lifestyle to stick.

During the first month, logging your start mealtime and last mealtime every day is helpful to keep you consistent. If you increase your fasting time or change your schedule later, continue to log for a month so that you can stay on plan. You can stop logging once your body starts to feel hungry at the new feeding time, and you do not get hungry after your last meal.

5. Maintain the schedule

Once you have fixed the time, keep the schedule consistent. Every now and then, your schedule or work may get in the way and disturb your fasting timing. That's okay. Get back on your feet and always strive to protect your fasting time.

Changing your eating schedule frequently confuses your digestive clocks. Your organs will be called upon to process food during an unusual eating window. Since it takes a few hours after processing for your digestive organs to get back into maintenance mode, there may not be enough maintenance period left before you feed them the next meal. If you want your entire digestive clock to function at its best, ensure that your feeding window is as consistent as possible.

As you maintain a consistent feeding window, your digestive clock will adjust within a few days. Your stomach will start to secrete digestive juices just before your usual eating time, you will experience hunger at the usual feeding time, and your pancreas will begin to produce insulin in anticipation of incoming food. After your last meal, you will not feel hungry anymore, because your brain has sent the signal to your stomach, liver, and other organs to start maintenance mode.

Ways to Lose Body Fat

The easiest way to start losing weight is by practicing time-restricted eating. If you are overweight, I guarantee that you will lose weight just by practicing time-restricted eating alone, without altering your diet and exercise.

When you are fasting, you are likely to eat less food in a day than when you are not fasting, thereby creating a caloric deficit.

Start with 12-hour fasting, and once you are comfortable, you can increase it to 13-hour, 14-hour, 15-hour, and 16-hour fasting to rapidly lose weight. The fat burning process increases sharply after 12 hours of fasting, making it incredibly useful to lose weight fast.

Increase the feeding duration if you wish, as you may be uncomfortable having to eat too much in one sitting, or it might be challenging to eat all your required calories within the feeding window. Once you are happy with your weight, you can go back to 12-hour fasting for maintenance.

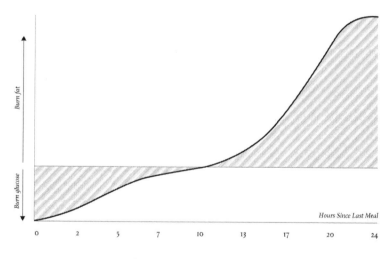

Glucose and Fat Burning Duration

Please note that you can do this without changing any other part of your routine. Introducing too many discomforts in one go may cause you to give up. In one to three weeks, you should start to notice your body slimming down. Look in the mirror and thank yourself for enduring the hardship.

One week after practicing time-restricted eating, I felt a significant improvement in my sleep. I began to dream again, something I did not remember having experienced for a long time. I began to fall asleep faster after lying down on the bed. I also felt that my usual anxiety subsided. It did not vanish, but it did recede. I did feel hungry almost every night, and that must be because I started with an 8-hour feeding window. I started with longer fasting hours and made myself suffer.

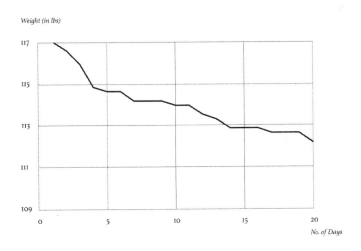

My Weight When Practicing Time-Restricted Eating

My weight at my scale dropped at a very rapid rate of 2.87 lbs during the first week, 1.32 lbs during the second week, 0.88 lbs during the third week, and then weight loss stalled. During my experiment, I dropped too much weight, more than what I wanted, so I later increased my feeding window by 1 hour. I still struggled to increase my weight. I later added one more extra meal, but still couldn't raise my weight. Adjusting my feeding window to be longer and increasing my meal intake got me to my suitable weight without feeling hunger at night.

Do not make yourself suffer by extending your fasting for too long every day and consuming as few calories as possible with the goal to accelerate the fat-burning rate. Aim to eat 25% fewer calories than your maintenance calories and do not create a calorie deficit that is too large.

Your body always wants to maintain homeostasis, the state in which the body thinks that it is already in its optimal condition. It does not like changes. There is an in-built mechanism to prevent you from dying of famine. When it senses that you have very small amounts of food available every day, your body is going to slow down all the internal processes to conserve precious energy. It uses only the energy needed to keep you alive. This brings down your basal metabolic rate, the number of calories burned at rest to keep your body functioning.

Over time, your body learns to use this small number of calories just to sustain your bodily functions. Your maintenance caloric requirement becomes lower, and the deficit that you trigger is no longer a deficit to your body. In the end, you stop losing weight. This is the main reason that crash diets do not work for the long term.

For men, aim to not go below 1,800 calories to avoid any side effects, and women should not go below 1,200. If you are not so obese, keep the calories deficit conservative and moderate. Otherwise, you will risk losing lean muscle, particularly with high training volume and intensity. It is fine, however, for obese people to be aggressive with their calorie deficit.

Now, while practicing time-restricted eating, you may ask what kind of diet you should follow. You are free to adopt any diet that already works for you. Many people swear by certain types of diets to lose weight, such as the Ketogenic diet or the Paleo diet. The problem with most kinds of diets is they are often too complicated and miserable to maintain in the long run. Resisting a particular type of food drains a lot of your willpower, which becomes worse if that food happens to be your favorite.

You need to keep challenging your self-control to resist carbohydrate food because the diet requires that you keep your carbohydrate intake to a certain number of grams per day. Your fasting protocol requires you to eat all your meals within four hours to drop as much weight as possible, and you sleep miserably hungry. Because the diets are too difficult to follow for the long term, and drain a lot of willpower, most people fail, binge-eat even more, and re-gain more weight than they lost on the diet.

If you have adopted and maintained any of these diets without problems, congratulations! Please continue with the diet and feel free to skip the remaining information in this chapter and resume the next chapter. If you have had no success with fat loss, read on.

Before we start, please note that this section aims to lose weight up to a healthy range. This is not the guide to get extremely low body fat percentages, such as that of a professional bodybuilder. For that, you need to seek expert advice and use advanced techniques that are not covered here.

Let's get to the basics of fat loss. The thermodynamic laws dictate that being in a state of calorie deficit makes you lose weight since your body cannot create energy out of nothing. Calorie deficit happens when the total calories you consume are *less than* the total calories used by your body.

It does not matter which diet you adopt, you will lose weight as long as it induces a calorie deficit, and you can adopt it as your routine. The same applies even if your diet consists of just junk food. If you can create a calorie deficit by eating junk food, you will lose weight. It comes down to how much you are willing to compromise your health to get the weight down on the scale.

When following any fat-loss diet, do not expect immediate results; your body needs time to melt the fat away. There is no way to spot-reduce fat in a specific part of your body such as your belly, as some products claim to be able to. Belly fat may be the last to be melted after the fat in other areas of your body is gone.

I recommend the following tips that worked well for me:

1. Occasionally, eat your favorite junk food and don't feel regretful

Yes, that's right. This gets to be my *top* recommendation. We all have our favorite childhood junk food that we like, or the MSG-loaded instant noodles that never fail to satisfy our taste buds. If you have been craving that, and you have the opportunity to eat them after a long time, please eat them to keep yourself sane without having even the slightest regret.

Do not make your diet miserable. Life is too good to let go of enjoyable food. Everyone knows they are bad, but eating them once in a while is fine, and then you can quickly get back on track.

I advocate a diet that makes you happy and is not miserable to follow. The more resistance you have to restrict any food that you like, the more energy is sapped from your willpower. This may eventually cause you to quit and return to your old routine. The cost of losing your willpower day by day far outweighs the temporary damage caused by eating that burger you've been craving for months. You can better use your willpower to build healthy routines and habits for your future goals.

As you continue to build better food control and prioritize whole food instead of junk food, you naturally make better food choices and want to avoid eating junk food. Over time, junk food doesn't look so appealing or appetizing anymore. You start to hate the feeling of your stomach being bloated after consuming high-sodium deep-fried chicken. We shall aim for this, rather than to stop eating junk food altogether when we start any fat loss program. As you venture into better eating habits, don't feel guilty if you wish to eat a particular food that you deem unhealthy from time to time. Enjoy the treat to the fullest.

2. Avoid sugar as much as you can

Sugar is addictive, encourages fat storage, causes insulin resistance, pre-diabetes, obesity, and inflammation. When your goal is to burn fat, consuming sugar does the opposite. It suppresses fat breakdown and makes your body insulin-resistant.

Removing sugar from your diet is going to be difficult. But, it is worth every effort for the long-term health benefit of making you insulin sensitive again after years of torture from sugary food. It is challenging to stay away from sugar, all the more so if you always eat out, because it is lurking in just about every product available at the supermarket. Practice reading product labels to check the content before purchasing anything.

As you cut sugar from your diet, you will experience sugar withdrawal symptoms. There will be an enormous craving for sugar during your first and even second weeks, but the cravings and withdrawal symptoms subside slowly. Now, it may be unrealistic to eliminate sugary food for your whole life. Consume sugary food occasionally, only when you crave one, but do it at day time when your insulin production peaks.

Fructose, which is contained in fruits, is sugar too. You may have a lifelong perception that consuming fruits is healthy. Fruits are loaded with vitamins, but they are just a different form of sugar. Consuming a lot of them inhibits fat loss. One thing to note about fructose is that only the liver can process fructose. In contrast, the whole body can use glucose for energy, including the liver. People often drink plenty of fruit juice without realizing how many calories and how much fructose it contains. This quickly disrupts blood sugar levels.

An important detail concerning our livers is that they can only hold about 100 grams of glycogen. The liver metabolizes fructose into glycogen and glucose, and any excess fructose which the liver can't hold will be converted to fat. To prevent any spillover to fat, the best time to consume fruit is in the morning when your liver tank is low, and after exercise, when the glucose in the liver has been depleted.

3. Always favor whole foods

It is challenging to avoid tasty processed food for the rest of your life. By all means, please enjoy it sporadically. If you are given a choice, always prioritize whole food. Whole food has a higher nutrient density compared to processed food, which means you get better nutrients with the same amount of calories.

4. Don't eliminate fat completely

Your body needs fat. People tout fat as a scary nutrient and some argue to avoid it at all costs. This is terrible advice and has misled us for decades. Our body needs fat to absorb certain vitamins and to protect vital organs. Furthermore, fat can be added to your starchy food to reduce its glycemic index. Eating fatty foods or oils with carbohydrates can slow the way glucose enters the bloodstream and prevent a spike in blood sugar levels.

Eat fat in moderation, and try to consume monounsaturated and polyunsaturated fats, instead of trans and saturated fats. Monounsaturated and polyunsaturated fats increase HDL cholesterol, the good cholesterol. Examples of food containing this kind of fats are olive oil, peanut oil, sesame oil, avocados, natural peanut butter, seeds, nuts, and fish oil.

Trans and saturated fats raise your LDL cholesterol, the bad cholesterol, clog your arteries, and raise your blood pressure. They are found in many processed or fast foods and animal fat. When consuming animal meat, always aim for lean meat.

5. Aim to eat a diverse range of food

Eat different types of food to obtain diverse nutrients from various foods. Do not eliminate animals' internal organs. They contain many nutrients that are hard to find in any other type of food. Consuming different types of food helps different populations of gut bacteria flourish and gives you better overall health.

6. Aim to consume protein in every meal

Our body requires more energy to metabolize protein. This is also known as the *thermic effect* of food. Adding protein at every meal causes your body to burn more calories.

Furthermore, while you are in a calorie deficit, you need to consume more protein than when you are in a calorie surplus to preserve your muscle mass. When you have fewer calories in the system, your body has the tendency to break down protein from the skeletal muscle to run the body's functions.

A CALORIE DEFICIT can be triggered by *consuming fewer calories* or *expending more calories,* or both. Time-restricted eating helps you consume fewer calories, while exercise helps you expend more calories. We will cover some notes about exercises that help with fat loss.

ANAEROBIC EXERCISE

Long after a strength training session is over, your body continues to use calories to restore muscle glycogen and rebuild damaged muscles. This effect is called Excess Post-exercise Oxygen Consumption (EPOC). The higher the intensity of the strength training session, the longer EPOC lasts.

Strength training promotes muscle-building and having a lot of muscle is the most efficient way to lose body fat. Muscle tissue burns calories at rest. Five kilograms of muscle tissue burns about fifty calories while at rest in a day. That is five potato chips. Imagine having your body burn an increased number of calories while sitting on your couch, doing nothing. Muscle also raises insulin sensitivity, which helps your body get more glucose stored into muscle cells instead of into fat.

You can continue to enjoy fat loss by practicing time-restricted eating alone, but without strength training, you will lose not only fat but also muscle. If your body thinks you don't need to use muscle, it is going to shed muscle as well, because maintaining muscle mass is an expensive operation as it is a metabolically active type of tissue. The result is what people call being "skinny fat," that is, having low muscle mass and also some fat on your body.

While you are in a calorie deficit, you will not be able to gain muscle. Your goal in lifting weights is simply to preserve muscle. Lift heavy weights with low repetitions, and limit lifting to failure because your recovery is going to be slow due to the reduced calorie intake.

If this is the first time you are lifting weights, you will gain some muscles quickly, also known as "newbie gain." This is because your muscles have never been shocked by the stimulation from strength training, and they compensate by building muscle mass at a faster rate. As you advance your training for an extended period, your sensitivity is getting reduced, so you need an even bigger stimulus to keep growing muscle mass.

Aerobic Exercise

Aerobic exercise is an optional choice. If your main purpose is building muscle, including aerobic exercise to your strength training program slows muscle growth.[9] If, however, your goal is to lose as much fat as possible, and building muscle is not your priority, then aerobic exercise can aid in the fat-burning process. Aerobics is an oxygen-dependent physical activity, and with the presence of oxygen, your body can mobilize fat.

Many theories state that doing cardio on an empty stomach after waking up can accelerate the fat-burning process since there is a low amount of carbohydrates in the system from the overnight sleep. If you don't do cardio on an empty stomach, you will need to exercise for nearly 20–30 minutes to deplete your carbohydrates first before your body starts to burn body fat.

With low carbohydrates in the system, however, you will soon experience a sudden loss of energy, and you won't be able to last long. When you exercise on an empty stomach, you increase the risk of hypoglycemia, low blood sugar, and if you do intense cardio, you increase catabolism, the breaking down of muscle cells. Your body will go through the process of gluconeogenesis to convert skeletal muscle to glucose, and you eventually lose more muscle.

When you perform cardio on a fed state, you have more fuel, and you can train harder and longer. Although you will burn less fat during the session, your body will continue to burn more fat after the session is over. You also preserve more muscle mass when you don't do cardio on an empty stomach. Over the course of a day, both fed and fasted cardio burn the same amount of fat.[10]

Let's understand how fat storage and carb storage are used. Your body burns both the calories from carbs and those from fat at a different pace based on your Maximum Heart Rate (MHR).

	Burned Carb	Burned Fat
65-70% MHR	40%	60%
70-75% MHR	50%	50%
75-80% MHR	65%	35%
80-85% MHR	80%	20%
85-90% MHR	90%	10%
90-95% MHR	95%	5%
100% MHR	100%	0%

Percentage of Carbohydrate and Fat Burned

Does this mean going with 65–70% of your MHR is the ultimate fastest way to burn fat? No. If you do High-Intensity Interval Training (HIIT) cardio, one that demands at least 75–80% MHR, you burn the same amount of fat compared to Light-Intensity Interval Training (LIIT) cardio for the same amount of time. Furthermore, as you burn more carbohydrates during HIIT cardio, your body will burn more fat after the exercise. Overall, the total calories expense is higher in HIIT, expediting your goal to a calorie deficit when you are trying to lose weight.

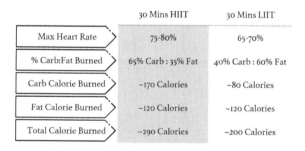

	30 Mins HIIT	30 Mins LIIT
Max Heart Rate	75-80%	65-70%
% Carb:Fat Burned	65% Carb : 35% Fat	40% Carb : 60% Fat
Carb Calorie Burned	~170 Calories	~80 Calories
Fat Calorie Burned	~120 Calories	~120 Calories
Total Calorie Burned	~290 Calories	~200 Calories

30 Minutes HIIT vs 30 Minutes LIIT

Intensity is the key. You save more time doing HIIT to burn more calories. If your only exercise is HIIT, aim not to exceed forty minutes, and do no more than four sessions per week, or you may get injured and risk overtraining. If you are already following a strength training program, adding HIIT exercises on top of it blunts your muscle recovery and increases your risk of overtraining. You should treat a HIIT session as another anaerobic session. Adding both HIIT and anaerobic exercise increases the training frequency and the risk of overtraining.

Adding a LIIT session on top of your weight-lifting program is fine and serves as an active recovery protocol to aid your muscle recovery. It is possible to perform HIIT in strength training, that is, by using lower weights, higher repetitions, and shorter rest duration.

COLD THERMOGENESIS

I would like to mention one more tool that could help you further speed up calorie expenditure, called *Cold Thermogenesis*. Exposing your body to cold temperatures increases brown fat. Brown fat, or Brown Adipose Tissue (BAT), burns calories when you expose your body to chilly temperatures. This process is called cold thermogenesis. Brown fat can be recruited from the infamous white fat inhabiting our bellies. Having higher levels of brown fat increases insulin sensitivity, lowers the risk of diabetes, increases fat-burning metabolism, and controls the blood sugar level.[11]

The conversion of white fat to brown fat accelerates when you expose your body to cool temperatures, such as submerging your body into cool water. Similar to exercise, cold thermogenesis at high intensity burns off muscle glycogen.

Once you empty the muscle glycogen, your muscle will be ready to absorb more glycogen when you eat carbohydrates.

An alternative practical way to expose your body to cold thermogenesis is by wearing a cooling vest that covers the shoulder and neck because these are the areas where brown fat is abundant. When you plan to indulge in cheat meals, use cold thermogenesis to your advantage.

Time it appropriately when you do this because you don't want to exhaust your glycogen stores very close to your strength training sessions. Give your body at least twelve hours to refill the glycogen stores before your strength training session begins. Do not do it right after your strength training, as it hampers muscle growth adaptation.[12]

WE HAVE LEARNED that time-restricted eating gets your eating clock in sync and fixes obesity at the same time. Now, we have completed the last lifestyle change that helps synchronize your circadian rhythm. If you have made all the preceding lifestyle changes, you'll experience a healthier circadian rhythm.

The next chapter unveils how to time your tasks throughout the day to harness your natural hormone fluctuations and be more productive.

5

OPTIMAL ROUTINE

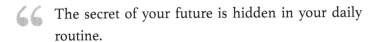 The secret of your future is hidden in your daily routine.

— MIKE MURDOCK

WE HAVE NOW REACHED THE FINAL CHAPTER OF THE BOOK AND learned the importance of a healthy circadian rhythm, good sleep quality, exercising, and practicing time-restricted eating. It's time to see what we can strategically do to make use of our body's circadian rhythms and the rising and falling of our hormone to be more productive.

Morning

WAKING HOUR

How you wake up is a crucial moment of the day. It sets you out with the right mood, which affects your productivity throughout the day.[1] You want to make sure you wake up in a happy mood. Using an alarm clock to wake up triggers a fight or flight response in your body, which induces stress. Your brain suddenly feels shocked and cannot quite work out what is going on.

It is not a pleasant experience you want to bear every working day. You want to feel refreshed and relaxed, not jump-started with a loud noise. When you are woken up while in a deep sleep, you will feel sleepy and groggy. Having an alarm set at a predefined time will probably wake you up at the wrong stage of your sleep, leaving you feeling dizzy and tired.

Fortunately, if you have your circadian rhythm in tune and a solid sleeping schedule, you will be able to wake up at your usual time without using an alarm clock. This ensures that you wake up happy, which is the first step towards gaining productive hours for the rest of your day.

Instead of using an alarm clock, use a smart bulb that can simulate daylight. It can be preset at your desired wake-up time to brighten up the room from low to full brightness. This allows you to wake up gently.

THE FIRST HOUR OF WAKING UP

- **Sunlight:** Upon waking up, have access to sunlight to reset your circadian clock, improve your mood, concentration, and melatonin secretion in the evening. It also decreases the impact of blue light on your melatonin at night. If you have no access to sunlight, use a bright light therapy device. Having less exposure to bright light during the day reduces your ability to make good decisions.

- **High willpower:** With your willpower bolstered by a full tank in the morning, you have more motivation to do what you have set yourself to do, and are very likely to stick to it. Use it to your advantage to do the most challenging task(s) that you have.

- **Exercise:** If you exercise in the morning, you can make use of the improved cognitive function from the increased BDNF during your working hours. Research reveals that morning exercise enhances the parasympathetic tone at night, as opposed to evening exercise.[2] This helps you to sleep better. Please note, however, that your muscle strength is not at its best in the morning, so if you are doing anaerobic exercise in the morning, you are more prone to injury. Do a more involved warm-up to reduce the risk of injury.

ENJOY YOUR (CHEAT) MEAL

If you are craving sugary, high-carbohydrate foods, plan to eat them in the morning. Your insulin response is at its peak in the morning and diminishes at night.[3] Your stomach can digest food at the fastest rate in the morning, and your gallbladder is efficient to produce bile to digest fat. Your fully powered digestive system is optimized to handle high-calorie and sugary food during the daytime.

Another time when you can enjoy your sweet treat is after exercise. After exercise, your body would have depleted your glycogen storage to some extent, and it is hungry to use the sugar to replenish the glycogen stores. Eating sweet food at that time is unlikely to get the sugar stored as fat.

CAFFEINE

A cup of coffee has been a morning pick-me-up for many people to wake their brains up. If you possess a robust circadian rhythm, you don't need coffee to keep you awake in the morning. In this case, consuming coffee first thing in the morning is only marginally beneficial.

Caffeine is a stimulant, and since you only have a chance to drink it before noon to avoid adverse effects to your sleep later on, you want to use it intentionally:

- As a pre-workout booster, caffeine stimulates the central nervous system to give you the extra jolt in your exercise.
- When you still need to work on something important in the morning after the initial focus and concentration wear off.

- When you need an extra boost to your brain power, such as during an examination.

If you consume coffee daily, the boosting effect of caffeine wears off as your body builds higher tolerances to caffeine. Your body will then require a more significant dose to give you a similar outcome. Once a month, schedule a week without coffee to desensitize yourself to the effects of caffeine.

If you do not drink coffee every day, you will notice the caffeine effect longer than people who drink coffee daily due to the higher sensitivity you have to caffeine.

Note: Mixing L-theanine supplement and caffeine at a 2:1 ratio —for example, 200 mg of L-theanine with 100 mg of caffeine or a cup of coffee—heightens your focus, and enhances your concentration and alertness.

SUPERCHARGED BRAIN

Between 10 a.m. and 2 p.m., the brain functions at its best and is most alert. Use these hours for learning, decision-making, solving complicated problems, focusing your attention, and making the best assessments. This timing happens to be when most people eat their lunch. If it is your lunchtime, take a short lunch in order not to waste much of your productive hours. One hour during this period is worth two or more hours during the late afternoon.

Afternoon

Afternoon Dip

Between 2:00 p.m. and 4:00 p.m., your sleep drive increases.[4] You will feel sluggish, noticeably if you ate a heavy lunch. This effect reduces your mental performance, analytical skills, and cognitive capability. It happens even if you did have a good night's sleep the night before, but it is worse if you did not.

To prevent the disruption of your sleep at night, avoid using coffee to survive the afternoon slump, as many people do. Taking a 45-minute nap can boost your mood and performance. However, do this with caution. We learned earlier that taking a nap lowers your sleep drive at night.

You can reduce the impact of the afternoon dip by:

- Doing some light physical activities after lunch.
- Exposing yourself to sunlight after your lunch for about 30 minutes.
- Reducing the portions of your food intake during these periods.

During your productive hours in the afternoon, ensure that your blood sugar level stays consistent. When you consume high-carbohydrate food, your insulin level will spike, and soon after that, it plummets, and you will temporarily feel tired, which hampers your work performance. If you eat high-carbohydrate food in the afternoon, aim to consume the following, which helps to balance sugar level:

- Green tea
- Lemon
- Grapefruit
- Linseed (flaxseed)
- Pistachios
- Apple cider vinegar
- Cinnamon
- Coffee (it aids to balance the blood sugar level, but is not an option past noon)
- Ginger
- Alpha-lipoic acid

If you can ride out these hours without your brain feeling foggy, you have essentially earned a few productive hours of the day that most people fail to use.

Optimize your working environment by doing the following:

- Gain access to natural light through windows near your desk to boost your mood and energy.
- Have plant(s) at your desk to oxygenate your brain and reduce your anxiety and stress level.
- Use an ergonomic chair and ensure the correct positioning of the monitor to avoid bending your back when working in front of a computer. A bad sitting posture strains your spinal discs.
- If you work in front of a computer monitor most of the time, wear computer eyeglasses to eliminate the problems caused by the glare from the screen, such as eye strains, blurred vision, and headaches.

- Declutter your workspace to promote focus and efficiency.
- Take frequent breaks to avoid sitting for long periods. After all, we are usually only able to concentrate on a task for ten to twenty-five minutes at a time.
- Use an aroma diffuser with scents such as lemon, peppermint, lavender, and chamomile to calm your mind.
- Eliminate as many interruptions as possible at your workplace. When you are interrupted, it takes almost twenty-three minutes to regain your full concentration. Schedule an uninterrupted block of time by placing a do-not-disturb sign at the entrance to your room, disconnecting your Internet, closing your email application, and setting your phone to silent when you are trying to produce high-quality work.

Late afternoon exercise

During the late afternoon, you can take advantage of your body's natural increase in muscle tone and strength to perform an anaerobic exercise like lifting weights or other forms of strength training. The added muscle tone during this time will help you lift more in the gym. Your heart rate is higher at this time, which helps distribute nutrients and oxygen throughout your body, meaning there is less chance of getting injured.

Evening

WIND-DOWN TIME

In the evening, give your body cues to start preparing for restful sleep.

1. Stop working

In the latter part of the day, the brain becomes less alert and attentive, and we are prone to making mistakes if we continue to use the brain to solve complicated problems. The brain's alertness level reverses as nighttime draws near, and it is primed for sleeping. When you have a tough decision to make in the evening, sleep on it, and make the decision the next day.

If you always burn the midnight oil to rush through your work, unfortunately, you are not doing your productivity any favors. It is an incorrect perception that working late equates to increased productivity. Getting sufficient sleep is the one that grants you higher performance at work.

No matter how hard you try, being deprived of sleep reduces your cognitive capability, which makes your work suffer. Any work you do when sleep-deprived will probably contain errors you'll need to fix later. Any decisions you make may not be sound. Working late to complete your task is not productive at all. You simply cannot force your brain to function optimally at this hour.

2. Stop eating

The circadian clocks of our digestive organs are not optimal at night, as they are preparing your body for maintenance and sleep.

.

- Eating closer to bedtime leaves the food, especially high-protein food, to be processed at a slower pace by the gut, and often triggers acid reflux if you go to sleep immediately afterward. The supine sleeping positions cause the high acids produced in the stomach to flow back to the esophagus.
- Late at night, saliva production decreases, and stomach acid production increases. When you eat at night, the excess stomach acid slowly travels to your mouth, but there is insufficient saliva in your mouth to help neutralize the acid, which could lead to tooth decay.
- Insulin response is slower at night than during the day. It takes longer for the body to clear up the spike in blood sugar after a meal, causing some of the excess sugar to be stored as fat, and as the glucose remains longer in the blood, you are more prone to develop insulin resistance. Melatonin produced at night reduces insulin production. This lowers the capacity of insulin to regulate blood sugar. If your blood sugar level drops while you are sleeping, you may be woken up from your sleep.
- Digesting food and absorbing its nutrients raises core body temperature. Your blood is diverted to your stomach and gut area to digest food and absorb

nutrients. Increasing core body temperature does not prime your body for sleep.

Food stays in the stomach for two to five hours before getting processed in the intestines. Once the food has left the stomach, your stomach reduces its acid production. You need to time your last meal to be at least two to five hours before your bedtime to ensure your stomach has completed the food digestion, reduced its acid production, and your core temperature has dropped before you sleep.

Having an empty stomach for an extended period before sleep gives you higher quality sleep, as your body does not require processing any food, the core temperature of the body is not elevated, and you have no chance of getting acid reflux.[5]

Aside from the impact on the circadian clock, you would have used up plenty of your willpower towards the end of the day. Your self-control is reduced a lot at night, and you have a higher risk of bingeing on junk food. All these issues disrupt your sleep quality.

However, if you must eat closer to bedtime, try to:

- Avoid high carbohydrate meals to minimize the sugar in the blood, since insulin production slows down in the evening. It will not be able to shuttle all the glucose in your blood, and the glucose will remain circulating in your bloodstream for a long time, most of which will be stored as fat, instead of used as energy. This promotes insulin resistance.
- Avoid sleeping or lying down immediately after your

dinner. Let gravity helps keep stomach acid in the stomach, reducing the chance of getting acid reflux.

- Perform mild physical activity after your last meal, such as walking your dog. Doing so helps digestion, reduces the blood sugar circulating in your blood, and lowers the risk of getting acid reflux.
- If it fits into your schedule, do your strength training before your last meal at night. After strength training, your body accelerates the absorption of glucose from your blood, which helps compensate for the reduced capacity of insulin at night.

3. Stop drinking

Timing your last heavy fluid intake of the day is important to ensure you are hydrated throughout your sleep but not woken up by a full bladder. A night of interrupted sleep is undesirable.

You should generally stop heavy water intake 2–3 hours before bedtime. Experiment with your last heavy fluid intake and keep track of the time you drink it to determine if you wake up with the urge to pass urine during your sleep. The goal is to find out the number of hours you can consume heavy water prior to your sleep without being woken up by a full bladder.

As you restrict your fluid intake closer to bedtime, you need to ensure you consume enough water during the day. After your last heavy water intake, you can sip a little water until bedtime. Place a glass of water at the side of your bed in case you wake up at night feeling thirsty. Take a sip and go back to sleep. Coping with thirst makes it more difficult to sleep.

If you drink alcohol, consider removing it from your diet. Alcohol impedes your sleep, in particular, if you drink it close to bedtime, by reducing the amount of your REM sleep, which is vital for consolidating your memories. People may think that drinking alcohol aids with fighting insomnia because it sends you to sleep faster, but they may not realize what it costs in the reduced amount of REM sleep. Alcohol also dehydrates you, and you will wake up thirsty during your sleep if you drink it within two to four hours before your bedtime.

4. Stop exercising

Intense exercise in the late evening elevates cortisol levels. Melatonin production is delayed when your cortisol level is high, which is detrimental to your sleep. The circadian clock may get confused and think it is daytime. Your body core temperature, heart rate, and breathing rate will elevate, which causes your sympathetic tone to increase, making it harder to fall asleep. Avoid exercising three hours before bed to allow sufficient time for your body to cool down.

If it is the only time you can work out, don't feel bad about the downsides. It is still better than not exercising at all. Paul Michael Levesque, who is better known as "Triple H," works out between 11 p.m. and midnight.

TIME TO GET CREATIVE

During the late evening, when your brain is tired, and the prefrontal cortex is not very active as you are winding down, your brain suppresses its reasoning part. This spurs creativity because you don't think about perfecting the idea you are thinking. It is a good moment to do creative work, like finding your business brand name or brainstorming the name of your new music album. Any idea in your head goes all out. You get the same effect when you are bored or daydreaming. Einstein's great ideas occurred most of the time when he was loafing around or taking a shower.

PRE-BED RITUAL

Adopt the following routine before going to bed:

1. Avoid exciting activities

Avoid any activity that arouses your brain, such as watching horror movies, reading terrifying news, solving mentally draining problems, or reviewing exciting trips close to bedtime. These activities raise your sympathetic tone. Replace them with activities that help your brain wind down and activate your parasympathetic tone, such as reading or listening to calming music.

2. Wear blue light blocking glasses

At least two hours before bedtime, wear blue light blocking glasses to reduce artificial light exposure after sunset and start stimulating the production of melatonin.

3. Consume a magnesium supplement

Magnesium has a calming and anti-stress effect in addition to reducing inflammation and lowering blood pressure levels. It induces calmness by activating the parasympathetic nervous system, which alleviates anxiety and depression.

Insufficient magnesium in your system makes it difficult for you to fall asleep. Surveys show that 75% of people have a deficiency of magnesium. High-stress levels from work and exercise further reduce the magnesium in our body through urination. If at night you experience restless leg syndrome, or the urge to move your legs as keeping them still feels uncomfortable, you may have a magnesium deficiency. Lack of magnesium also causes leg cramps at night.

Consume magnesium between one to two hours before bedtime to help you sleep. Adult females need about 310 to 320 mg of magnesium per day, while adult males need 400 to 420 mg per day. Higher doses of magnesium, more than 600 mg, may keep you up at night instead of helping you sleep. Always begin with a lower dose and see how your body reacts. Remember that you may have already obtained some amount of magnesium from your food.

There is a broad range of choices for magnesium. You can consider either magnesium citrate or magnesium glycinate. Both work well for better sleep. Magnesium citrate works by binding water into your intestine, which also softens your stool. Aim to drink plenty of water when consuming this type of magnesium to avoid dehydration. As you may have consumed some magnesium from your diet, start with a smaller dose until your stool becomes watery. Magnesium glycinate, on the other hand, does not soften the stool, but it does cause the same calming effect as magnesium citrate does to help with sleep.

4. Meditate

Meditation quiets your mind and enhances your inner peace. These are the ingredients for anxiety-free sleep. Ten to twenty minutes of meditation before bed eases the tension you accumulated throughout the day.

Meditation also increases the production of serotonin, a "feel-good" neurotransmitter, decreases blood pressure, and decreases heart rate, which sets the stage for better sleep.

5. Use a Pulsed Electromagnetic Field (PEMF) device

When you are relaxed, your brain produces higher *Alpha* brainwaves, and when you are sleeping, your brain produces higher *Theta* brainwaves. It is sometimes difficult for your brain to go into these states if you are leading a stressful life. You can use PEMF technology to entrain your brain to enter into the desired state. It emits the correct frequency to encourage your brain to align to that frequency and get into *Alpha* or *Theta* state almost immediately. PEMF is a drug-free therapy that has been studied for at least twenty years to be safe for brain entrainment.

6. Use a Cranial Electrotherapy Stimulation (CES) device

If you are suffering from insomnia, anxiety, and depression, you can invest in a CES device. It has been used for decades to alleviate insomnia, anxiety, and depression.[6] A CES device uses a pair of wet sponges to send small currents to the brain to stabilize your mood by stimulating the production of feel-good neurotransmitter inhibitors, serotonin, and dopamine. Daily consumption of caffeine or stimulants depletes serotonin over time. Instead of resorting to taking medication to tackle insomnia, CES is an alternative solution without any recorded side effects, including addiction.

What's Next?

We have completed the steps to optimize your routine around your circadian clock. The final thing that can help you exceed the ceiling of your current performance is improving your neuroplasticity. Your brain is morphing every moment, and it is still forming brain cell connections even after you are long past your childhood. Your brain evolves into a better or worse version of itself based on what stimulus you give it.

If you stop learning new things and always engage in less effortful cognitive exercises, your brain cells will start to degenerate, causing a deterioration of your skills. You will suffer a loss of brain cells, your brain will lose some of its function, and you will begin to form bad habits much more quickly. If you often stimulate your brain with negative thoughts, such as through constant worrying and stress, it could lead to anxiety or mental illness over time. This is called neuroplasticity. Similar to the muscles of your body, you can improve your brain's neuroplasticity by exercising the habits listed below:

- Challenging your brain to solve complicated problems.
- Learning new skills, musical instruments, or languages.
- Reading books.
- Having adequate sleep.
- Meditation.
- Fasting.
- Physical exercise.
- Brain entrainment.

Improving neuroplasticity is a way to upgrade your brain continuously, and the only limitation is your lifespan. I covered a detailed plan and strategy to maximize your brain plasticity in *Peak Brain Plasticity*.

CONCLUSION

You have learned the importance of a fixed sleeping schedule, a consistent eating pattern, and integrating exercise into your routine to restore a healthy circadian rhythm. All these will make it possible for you to manage your tasks around the optimal time of your day and amplify your productivity considerably. You can continue to push through plateaus by practicing habits that enhance your neuroplasticity.

Put an effort to make these your way of life. You will see the optimal, rejuvenated version of yourself, and you will thank yourself for the progress you can achieve in your life.

Now, put what you have learned into action. Having knowledge without putting it into action is futile.

- If you are an employer, recognize that you'd be better off having your staff go home for restorative sleep and resume their work the next day than having them rush work at night with more errors, while sabotaging their health in later years.

- If you are a parent, don't encourage your children to study late at night for examinations. If they do, they will perform with reduced cognitive function during the test.
- If you are a busy professional, spend time exercising to boost your performance.
- If you are a dieter and have not been able to lose weight despite trying your best to snack on healthy food, integrate time-restricted eating into your routine.

My wish and the reason I wrote this book is that people will realize they can reach the best of their abilities by harnessing the power of their own circadian rhythm. Now, spread the message to your friends and family members about how important it is to make time to exercise, practice a consistent sleeping schedule, and incorporate time-restricted eating to function at their best. If any of them is in poor health, don't give up just yet. A robust circadian rhythm restores the balance in your body and fends off many critical diseases. It could at least alleviate, if not cure, the illness.

Thank you for reading the book.

KEEP IN TOUCH

If this book benefits you, would you please take a moment to write a review on Amazon? I would love to read your comments. It would mean a lot to me hearing directly from readers like you.

Keep in touch with me at said@saidhasyim.com and let me know if you need any help.

If you wish to be notified of my next book update, sign up to my mailing list at https://www.saidhasyim.com/contact

ALSO BY SAID HASYIM

ABOUT THE AUTHOR

Said Hasyim is a certified IT project manager with an obsession for finding the best ways to maximize his productivity. After half a decade of arduous self-experimentation and research into bio-hacks, willpower, lifestyle changes, neuroplasticity, and sleep routines, Said discovered various methods to improve his productivity. Now, he hopes to share his findings with his readers in his *Peak Productivity book series* to unleash their inner potential. Find out more about Said at www.saidhasyim.com.

DISCLAIMER

This book contains advice and information relating to health care. It should be used to supplement rather than replace the advice of your doctor or another trained health professional. If you know or suspect you have a health problem, it is recommended that you seek your physician's advice before embarking on any medical program or treatment. All efforts have been made to assure the accuracy of the information contained in this book as of the date of publication. The author disclaims liability for any medical outcomes that may occur as a result of applying the methods suggested in this book.

NOTES

1. Circadian Clock

1. University of California - Irvine. (2019, May 30). Circadian clocks: Body parts respond to day and night independently from brain, studies show. *ScienceDaily*. Retrieved February 9, 2021 from www.sciencedaily.com/releases/2019/05/190530141443.htm
2. Schroeder, A. M., & Colwell, C. S. (2013). How to fix a broken clock. *Trends in pharmacological sciences*, 34(11), 605–619. https://doi.org/10.1016/j.tips.2013.09.002

2. Master Your Sleep to Master Your Performance

1. Stats: 51% of adults worldwide don't get enough sleep. (2018, August 8). Retrieved from https://www.travelagentcentral.com/running-your-business/stats-51-adults-worldwide-don-t-get-enough-sleep
2. RAND Corporation. (2016, November 30). Lack of sleep costing US economy up to $411 billion per year. ScienceDaily. Retrieved July 13, 2019 from www.sciencedaily.com/releases/2016/11/161130130826.htm
3. Hafner, M., Stepanek, M., Taylor, J., Troxel, W. M., & van Stolk, C. (2017). Why sleep matters—the economic costs of insufficient sleep: A cross-country comparative analysis. Rand health quarterly, 6(4), 11.
4. Kwok, C. S., et al. (2018). Self-reported sleep duration and quality and cardiovascular disease and mortality: A dose-response meta-analysis. Journal of the American Heart Association, 7(15), 1. https://doi.org/10.1161/jaha.118.008552
5. Takeuchi, H., Taki, Y., Nouchi, R. *et al.* Shorter sleep duration and better sleep quality are associated with greater tissue density in the brain. *Sci Rep* **8**, 5833 (2018). https://doi.org/10.1038/s41598-018-24226-0
6. Uppsala University. (2016, August 10). Plenty of light during daytime reduces the effect of blue light screens on night sleep. ScienceDaily. Retrieved May 16, 2020 from www.sciencedaily.com/releases/2016/08/160810104246.htm

7. Garaulet, M., Qian, J., Florez, J. C., Arendt, J., Saxena, R., & Scheer, F. (2020). Melatonin effects on glucose metabolism: Time to unlock the controversy. *Trends in endocrinology and metabolism: TEM, 31*(3), 192–204. https://doi.org/10.1016/j.tem.2019.11.011

8. Ko, Y., & Lee, J. Y. (2018). Effects of feet warming using bed socks on sleep quality and thermoregulatory responses in a cool environment. *Journal of physiological anthropology, 37*(1), 13. https://doi.org/10.1186/s40101-018-0172-z

9. Tähkämö, L., Partonen, T., & Pesonen, A. K. (2019). Systematic review of light exposure impact on human circadian rhythm. *Chronobiology international, 36*(2), 151–170. https://doi.org/10.1080/07420528.2018.1527773

10. Lillehei, A. S., & Halcon, L. L. (2014b). A systematic review of the effect of inhaled essential oils on sleep. The Journal of Alternative and Complementary Medicine, 20(6), 441–451. https://doi.org/10.1089/acm.2013.0311

11. Strøm-Tejsen, P., Zukowska, D., Wargocki, P., & Wyon, D. P. (2015). The effects of bedroom air quality on sleep and next-day performance. Indoor Air, 26(5), 679–686. https://doi.org/10.1111/ina.12254

12. Zhao, J., Tian, Y., Nie, J., Xu, J., & Liu, D. (2012). Red light and the sleep quality and endurance performance of Chinese female basketball players. Journal of Athletic Training, 47(6), 673–678. https://doi.org/10.4085/1062-6050-47.6.08

3. We Are Born to Move

1. World Health Organization. (2005). World health day: Sedentary lifestyle: A global public health problem. Retrieved from https://www.who.int/docstore/world-health-day/2002/fact_sheets4.en.shtml

2. Hower, I. M., Harper, S. A., & Buford, T. W. (2018). Circadian rhythms, exercise, and cardiovascular health. Journal of Circadian Rhythms, 16(1), 3. https://doi.org/10.5334/jcr.164

3. Pronk, N. P., Martinson, B., Kessler, R. C., Beck, A. L., Simon, G. E., & Wang, P. (2004). The association between work performance and physical activity, cardiorespiratory fitness, and obesity. Journal of Occupational and Environmental Medicine, 46(1), 19–25. https://doi.org/10.1097/01.jom.0000105910.69449.b7

4. Goekint, M., De Pauw, K., Roelands, B., Njemini, R., Bautmans, I., Mets, T., & Meeusen, R. (2010). Strength training does not influence serum brain-derived neurotrophic factor. European Journal of Applied Physiology, 110(2), 285–293. https://doi.org/10.1007/s00421-010-1461-3

5. Marston, K. J., Newton, M. J., Brown, B. M., Rainey-Smith, S. R., Bird, S., Martins, R. N., & Peiffer, J. J. (2017). Intense resistance exercise increases peripheral brain-derived neurotrophic factor. Journal of Science and Medicine in Sport, 20(10), 899–903. https://doi.org/10.1016/j.jsams.2017.03.015

6. Heaney, J. L. J., Carroll, D., & Phillips, A. C. (2014). Physical activity, life events stress, cortisol, and DHEA: Preliminary findings that physical activity may buffer against the negative effects of stress. Journal of Aging and Physical Activity, 22(4), 465–473. https://doi.org/10.1123/japa.2012-0082

7. Schoenfeld, B. (2012). The M.A.X. Muscle Plan (First ed.). Champaign, United States: Human Kinetics, Inc.

8. Aragon, A. A., & Schoenfeld, B. J. (2013). Nutrient timing revisited: Is there a post-exercise anabolic window?. *Journal of the International Society of Sports Nutrition*, *10*(1), 5. https://doi.org/10.1186/1550-2783-10-5

9. Ferguson-Stegall, L., et al. (2011). Postexercise carbohydrate–protein supplementation improves subsequent exercise performance and intracellular signaling for protein synthesis. Journal of Strength and Conditioning Research, 25(5), 1210–1224. https://doi.org/10.1519/jsc.0b013e318212db21

10. Pascoe DD, Costill DL, Fink WJ, Robergs RA, Zachwieja JJ. Glycogen resynthesis in skeletal muscle following resistive exercise. Med Sci Sports Exerc. 1993;25(3):349–354.

11. Graves, J., Pollock, M., Leggett, S., Braith, R., Carpenter, D., & Bishop, L. (1988). Effect of reduced training frequency on muscular strength. International Journal of Sports Medicine, 09(05), 316–319. https://doi.org/10.1055/s-2007-1025031

12. Methenitis S. (2018). A brief review on concurrent training: From laboratory to the field. Sports (Basel, Switzerland), 6(4), 127. https://doi.org/10.3390/sports6040127

13. Venuto, T. (2013). Burn the fat, feed the muscle: Transform your body forever using the secrets of the leanest people in the world (Revised ed.). New York City, United States: Harmony.

14. Youngstedt, S. D., Kline, C. E., Elliott, J. A., Zielinski, M., Devlin, T. M., & Moore, T. A. (2016). Circadian phase-shifting effects of bright light, exercise, and bright light + exercise. Journal of Circadian Rhythms, 14(1), 2. DOI: http://doi.org/10.5334/jcr.137

4. Eat How We Ate

1. Obesity and overweight. (2020, April 1). Retrieved from https://www.who.int/news-room/fact-sheets/detail/obesity-and-overweight
2. Goettler, A., Grosse, A., & Sonntag, D. (2017). Productivity loss due to overweight and obesity: A systematic review of indirect costs. BMJ open, 7(10), e014632. https://doi.org/10.1136/bmjopen-2016-014632
3. Panda, S. (2018). The circadian code: Lose weight, supercharge your energy, and transform your health from morning to midnight (First ed.). Pennsylvania, United States: Rodale Books.
4. Varady, K. A., Bhutani, S., Church, E. C., & Klempel, M. C. (2009). Short-term modified alternate-day fasting: A novel dietary strategy for weight loss and cardioprotection in obese adults. The American Journal of Clinical Nutrition, 90(5), 1138–1143. https://doi.org/10.3945/ajcn.2009.28380
5. Ho, K. Y., Veldhuis, J. D., Johnson, M. L., Furlanetto, R., Evans, W. S., Alberti, K. G., & Thorner, M. O. (1988). Fasting enhances growth hormone secretion and amplifies the complex rhythms of growth hormone secretion in man. Journal of Clinical Investigation, 81(4), 968–975. https://doi.org/10.1172/jci113450
6. Longer daily fasting times improve health and longevity in mice. (2018, September 6). Retrieved from https://www.nia.nih.gov/news/longer-daily-fasting-times-improve-health-and-longevity-mice
7. Wilkinson, M. J., Manoogian, E. N. C., Zadourian, A., Lo, H., Fakhouri, S., Shoghi, A., ... Taub, P. R. (2020). Ten-hour time-restricted eating reduces weight, blood pressure, and atherogenic lipids in patients with metabolic syndrome. Cell Metabolism, 31(1), 92-104.e5. https://doi.org/10.1016/j.cmet.2019.11.004
8. Li, L., Wang, Z., & Zuo, Z. (2013). Chronic intermittent fasting improves cognitive functions and brain structures in mice. PloS one, 8(6), e66069. https://doi.org/10.1371/journal.pone.0066069
9. Hickson, R. C. (1980). Interference of strength development by simultaneously training for strength and endurance. European Journal of Applied Physiology and Occupational Physiology, 45(2–3), 255–263. https://doi.org/10.1007/bf00421333
10. Schoenfeld, B. J., Aragon, A. A., Wilborn, C. D., Krieger, J. W., & Sonmez, G. T. (2014). Body composition changes associated with fasted versus non-fasted aerobic exercise. Journal of the International Society of Sports Nutrition, 11(1), 54. https://doi.org/10.1186/s12970-014-0054-7

11. Stanford KI, Middelbeek RJ, Townsend KL, et al. (2012). Brown adipose tissue regulates glucose homeostasis and insulin sensitivity. Journal of Clinical Investigation, 123(1), 215–223. https://doi.org/10.1172/jci62308

12. Roberts, L. A., Raastad, T., Markworth, J. F., Figueiredo, V. C., Egner, I. M., Shield, A., Cameron-Smith, D., Coombes, J. S., & Peake, J. M. (2015). Post-exercise cold water immersion attenuates acute anabolic signalling and long-term adaptations in muscle to strength training. The Journal of physiology, 593(18), 4285–4301. https://doi.org/10.1113/JP270570

5. Optimal Routine

1. Rothbard, N. P., & Wilk, S. L. (2011). Waking up on the right or wrong side of the bed: Start-of-workday mood, work events, employee affect, and performance. Academy of Management Journal, 54(5), 959–980. https://doi.org/10.5465/amj.2007.0056

2. Yamanaka, Y., Hashimoto, S., Takasu, N. N., Tanahashi, Y., Nishide, S., Honma, S., & Honma, K. (2015). Morning and evening physical exercise differentially regulate the autonomic nervous system during nocturnal sleep in humans. American Journal of Physiology-Regulatory, Integrative and Comparative Physiology, 309(9), R1112–R1121. https://doi.org/10.1152/ajpregu.00127.2015

3. Carroll, K. F., & Nestel, P. J. (1973). Diurnal variation in glucose tolerance and in insulin secretion in man. Diabetes, 22(5), 333–348. https://doi.org/10.2337/diab.22.5.333

4. Slama, H., Deliens, G., Schmitz, R., Peigneux, P., & Leproult, R. (2015). Afternoon nap and bright light exposure improve cognitive flexibility post lunch. PloS one, 10(5), e0125359. https://doi.org/10.1371/journal.pone.0125359

5. Crispim, C. A., Zimberg, I. Z., dos Reis, B. G., Diniz, R. M., Tufik, S., & de Mello, M. T. (2011b). Relationship between food intake and sleep pattern in healthy individuals. Journal of Clinical Sleep Medicine, 07(06), 659–664. https://doi.org/10.5664/jcsm.1476

6. Feusner, J. D., Madsen, S., Moody, T. D., Bohon, C., Hembacher, E., Bookheimer, S. Y., & Bystritsky, A. (2012). Effects of cranial electrotherapy stimulation on resting state brain activity. Brain and Behavior, 2(3), 211–220. https://doi.org/10.1002/brb3.45

Made in the USA
Middletown, DE
21 February 2021